D1557288

The Sword of Laban: Joseph Smith, Jr. and the Dissociated Mind

The Sword of Laban: Joseph Smith, Jr. and the Dissociated Mind

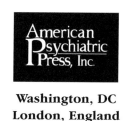

William D. Morain, M.D.

American Psychiatric Press, Inc.

Washington, DC
London, England

Copyright © 1998 American Psychiatric Press, Inc.
ALL RIGHTS RESERVED
Manufactured in the United States of America on acid-free paper
First Edition
01 00 99 98   4 3 2 1

American Psychiatric Press, Inc.
1400 K Street, N.W., Washington, DC   20005
www.appi.org

Library of Congress Cataloging-in-Publication Data
Morain, William D., 1942–
    The sword of Laban : Joseph Smith, Jr. and the dissociated mind   /
William D. Morain. — 1st ed.
        p.   cm
    Includes bibliographical references and index.
    ISBN 0-88048-864-6 (alk. paper)
    1. Smith, Joseph, 1805–1844—Mental health. 2. Post-traumatic stress
disorder—Patients—United States—Biography. 3. Dissociative dis-
orders—Patients—United States—Biography. 4. Church of Jesus Christ of
Latter-Day Saints—Biography. 5. Prophets (Mormon theology)—United
States—Biography. 6. Mormons—United States—Biography. I. Title.
    [DNLM: 1. Smith, Joseph, 1805–1844. 2. Stress disorders, Post-
Traumatic—case studies. 3. Dissociative Disorders—case studies.
4. Famous Persons. 5. Christianity—biography. WM 170 M827s 1998]
BX8695.S6M 59 1998
289.3′092—dc21
[B]
DNLM/DLC
for Library of Congress   97-25435
                                                                                CIP

British Library Cataloguing in Publication Data
A CIP record is available from the British Library.

***To Anne and Peter**
who taught me of fatherhood*

Contents

(f)oreword

r. Morain's remarkable psychological study of Joseph
Smith, Jr., the founder of Mormonism, will be of interest
to a wide spectrum of readers, as social history, as religious biography, as an account of the dissociative elements in poetic and
spiritual genius, or simply as a gripping portrait of an ill-fated and
tragic man. The volume, moreover, has a special relevance for
contemporary psychiatric clinicians, who are currently undergoing a major transition in their theoretical and practical approach
to psychiatric illness. This last aspect of Dr. Morain's book can
best be appreciated against the background of the brief overview
of the rise and fall of psychodynamic psychiatry that follows.

When Freud (in concert with his erstwhile colleague Josef
Breuer) commented in 1893, "Hysterics suffer mainly from reminiscences,"[1] he entered the lists of a controversy over the nature
and origin of psychological dissociation and its role in the etiology of psychiatric disorders that has intermittently dogged psychiatric theory and practice ever since. Although Freud's dictum was
uttered in confirmation of Janet's earlier clinical discovery of the

---

[1] Breuer J, Freud S: "On the Psychical Mechanism of Hysterical Phenomena:
Preliminary Communication" (1893), in *Standard Edition of the Complete
Psychological Works of Sigmund Freud*, Vol. 2. Translated and edited by
Strachey J. London, Hogarth Press, 1955, pp. 1–17.

central role played by memories of traumatic experiences in the production of a wide variety of psychiatric symptoms,[2] there were from the start significant differences in the respective formulations of the two men regarding the underlying mechanisms of symptom formation.[3]

In Janet's formulation, the concept of dissociation played a major role. Every individual, Janet proposed, is endowed at birth with a basic quantum of mental energy that serves to bind together that individual's psychological functions (memory, feeling, volition, etc.) in a coordinated whole under the control of the personal self, or ego. If the individual suffers a traumatic experience, the resulting emotional arousal so depletes that mental energy that the ability of the ego to maintain an integrated structure is severely compromised. As a consequence, the individual is unable to bind the memories of the traumatic event to the rest of his or her psychic structure; they become dissociated from that structure and now persist outside of the conscious awareness and control of the ego. However, although thus rendered unconscious, the dissociated memories nevertheless continue to affect the individual's functioning by producing consciously experienced ego-alien symptoms whose character is determined by the nature of the underlying memory images.

Freud, as noted earlier, concurred with Janet's delineation of the pathogenic role of traumatic memories, but he differed significantly in his formulation of the pathological processes that rendered them unconscious. The exclusion of such memories from consciousness, Freud proposed, occurs because the ego *actively* banishes them from conscious awareness and prevents their voluntary recall in order to protect itself from experiencing the painful affects associated with the memories of the trauma itself. That is, Freud proposed a model of symptom formation that

[2] Janet P: *l'Automatisme psychologique*. Paris, Félix Alcan, 1889.

[3] Nemiah JC: "Early Concepts of Trauma, Dissociation, and the Unconscious: Their History and Current Implications," in *Trauma, Memory, and Dissociation*. Edited by Bremner D, Marmar CR. Washington, DC, American Psychiatric Press, 1998, pp. 1–26.

involved a conflict of opposing psychological forces that ema-
nated from the components of a complex psychic structure and
were maintained in a dynamic equilibrium within that structure.
Janet, it may be said, adhered to a *deficit model* of mental function in which mental elements were lost to conscious awareness
and control when they underwent dissociation in a passive
falling-away from an ego too weak to maintain them in a unified
psychic structure. Freud, on the other hand, viewed dissociation
as resulting from the repression of traumatic memories and their
associated affects by an ego strong enough to exclude them from
conscious awareness and to maintain them in an unconscious
state. Freud, in other words, proposed a *conflict model* of psychopathology that has been the basis of psychodynamic theory and
practice ever since.

It should, moreover, be noted that in addition to emphasizing
the dynamic nature of psychogenesis, Freud differed from Janet
in abandoning the notion (prominent in Janet's formulations)
that psychologically traumatic events, especially in childhood,
were the primary cause of psychological dysfunction. Freud's
shifting view of etiology arose from his continued clinical investigations, which demonstrated that patients' apparent memories
of childhood traumas, in particular those that were sexual in nature, were in fact memories of childhood fantasies and feelings associated with disturbances in the phases of early psychological
growth and development. Adult psychological disorders, it became apparent, resulted from unresolved, *internally* derived psychic conflicts, not from distortions produced by *externally*
experienced traumatic events.

As the discipline of psychiatry developed during the early decades of the twentieth century, especially in the United States, the
Freudian dynamic model became the dominantly guiding theme in
psychiatric theory and practice, while Janet's conceptual approach
faded into obscurity. However, in the face of the meteoric rise of
biological psychiatry in the second half of this century, the influence of dynamic principles has dramatically waned, and dynamic
psychiatry, if it persists at all, is now merely one of a multitude of
"tracks" in psychiatric clinical centers and training programs.

It is, therefore, a matter of considerable interest that psychiatric clinicians are currently developing a renewed concern with the psychogenic aspects of psychiatric illness. Stimulated by an apparent increase in the incidence of both multiple personality disorder (now reclassified as dissociative identity disorder) and posttraumatic stress disorder (PTSD), investigators and clinicians alike have focused their attention on the etiological role of pathogenic trauma and the resulting dissociative processes that are a central feature of each clinical condition. In so doing, they have revived the century-old traumatic model of symptom formation that, as we have seen, invoked dissociated traumatic memories as the central etiological factor.

This return to an earlier formulation confronts modern clinicians with at least two conceptual and practical problems. It has, in the first place, stimulated a major and as yet unresolved controversy regarding the validity and etiological significance of memories of childhood sexual abuse recovered by adult patients in the course of psychotherapy. The veridicality of such memories is especially called into question when the occurrence of the alleged abuse has not been corroborated by independent evidence. Second, the current emphasis on the etiological role of external trauma, although it underscores a vital aspect of psychogenesis never fully appreciated after Freud abandoned it, has itself led modern clinicians to overlook the central importance for the production of psychiatric illness of the internally derived psychological conflicts resulting from distortions of early growth and development.

It is a central virtue of Dr. Morain's approach to the vicissitudes of Joseph Smith's history that he has avoided both of those obstacles to clinical understanding. He has, in the first place, exhumed from contemporary documents an objective account of the details of an overwhelmingly painful surgical procedure endured by Joseph Smith at the age of seven, a traumatic event whose subsequent reverberations Dr. Morain traces in the repetitive patterns of behavior and fantasies of Smith's adult life. Furthermore, Dr. Morain goes beyond the pathogenic effect of the traumatic episode to demonstrate how the horrifying *real* events of the surgery combined with the developmental phase-specific *fantasies* of a seven-year-old boy to bring about a permanent pathological distortion of Joseph Smith's entire early psychological growth and development, with significant consequences for his subsequent adult psychological functioning. In so doing, the author effectively combines the traumatic and dynamic models of symptom formation in a way that avoids the conceptual polarization potentially damaging to psychiatric theory and practice.

Finally, Dr. Morain's rich and skillfully crafted history of a complex and deeply troubled human life reminds us of the invaluable contribution to psychiatric understanding of the single case report, a method of clinical study that has now been largely crowded off the stage by the modern propensity for standardized interviews, patient self-report questionnaires, and the statistical manipulations of the data derived from them. The latter methods of study are, of course, invaluable for the scientific determination of the classification and distribution of psychiatric disorders and for their correlation with a variety of relevant variables. But the complementary task of exploring and delineating the unconscious conflicts that shape human behavior, relationships, and psychopathology can be accomplished only by combining the extended study of one human being by another with a presentation of the results in a richly detailed clinical biography, as Dr. Morain so gracefully and sensitively demonstrates in the work that follows.

John C. Nemiah, M.D.
Professor of Psychiatry,
Dartmouth Medical School;
Professor of Psychiatry Emeritus,
Harvard Medical School

Preface

*P*eter loves fairy tales—not the sanitized Disney versions, but the uncensored variety where folks get what they deserve. One night at a particularly late hour when I found myself thumbing through our unabridged Grimm for an especially short fairy tale, I ran across a two-pager entitled "The Lamb and the Fish." As there aren't many tales in Grimm that tell of an affectionate brother and sister, Peter's wide five-year-old eyes were especially smiling that night. The story told of the replacement of a loving mother by a hateful stepmother who changes the boy into a fish and the girl into a lamb. When guests arrive at the castle, the stepmother, seeing the opportunity to be rid of her stepdaughter altogether, orders the cook to feed the lamb to the visitors. The bound lamb-sister watches in terror as the cook brazenly sharpens his butcher knife while the fish-brother swims over to comfort the lamb in mutual condolence. When the cook discovers the two conversing, he correctly surmises that they have been bewitched by the mistress and hands them over to the children's former nurse for protection, substituting another animal for dinner. The nurse guesses the children's identity and arranges to have the spell broken to secure the children's safety.

"What is this?" I asked, trying to feign insult. "There was no daddy in that story. Where do you suppose the daddy was?" Without the least hesitation, Peter answered disdainfully, "The *cook* was the daddy."

Having carefully digested Bruno Bettelheim's sensitive psychoanalytic study of fairy tales,[1] I could probably have reached the same conclusion about the "daddy's" identity myself after a few minutes' reflection, but Peter knew instantly. The character acting on the controlling mother's command, the threatening one who would maim and kill the child, the one with the big, sharp knife—there was nothing difficult about that identity for an attentive five-year-old.

Bettelheim, a psychoanalyst with special interest in children, made a convincing case that fairy tales help a child to experience the common mortal fears shared by all his or her peers by allowing him or her to express those fears in the world of imagination. Thus those unspeakably threatening fantasies already lurking in Peter's mind may be shared with simpletons, giants, and princesses in ways that assure him that the world has a sense of order and fairness. His rapt attention has been such confirmation for me of Bettelheim's wisdom that I have made certain that a different fairy tale is served up at each bedtime.

The chances are good that I could have answered the "daddy" question just as quickly in my own kindergarten year, even though I have no recall for such notions. Five-year-olds, it seems, have a different way of knowing. And the fact that Peter will have to read Bettelheim's work in a couple of decades to understand what he now knows, but soon will not, is the reason my book and others like it are written.

Of course what Peter knows about the cook will not be forgotten in the sense of the wag who paraphrased Senator Howard Baker's famous question about the Watergate scandal, "What did the president know, and when did he stop knowing it?" Peter's ceasing to know will instead be a kind of metamorphosis of his notions about the cook from his world of immediacy to his mind's shadow world, where these notions can be neither remembered nor recognized. But in the transformation, this body of knowledge will become something far more significant, a kind of hid-

---

[1] Bettelheim B: *The Uses of Enchantment: The Meaning and Importance of Fairy Tales.* New York, Vintage Books, 1975, pp. 3–6.

den force in his behavior, as it was in his daddy's behavior and his daddy's daddy's before him.

It is axiomatic that this nonrational world of childhood fantasy can never be fully correlated with all nuances of adult behavior. However, many such themes may be strongly suspected, especially when horrifying events in childhood reinforce and distort those fantasies. Especially in biographical studies, knowledge of such early events may give partial answers to historian Herbert Muller's lament that "the main problem is not so much to fill in the many gaps of our factual knowledge as to make sense out of the vast deal that we do know."[2]

I have spent more than two decades in the training and academic practice of plastic and reconstructive surgery. This particular niche in the world of therapeutics is one which provides a special vantage point for observing the short- and long-term reactions of adults and children to deformity and to their own encounters with medical treatment for such misfortune. Sometimes psychiatric consultation has been needed for assistance in my understanding and management of such cases. But as Yogi Berra once remarked, "Sometimes you can observe a lot by just looking."

Child psychiatrist Lenore Terr has written, "A whole life can be shaped by an old trauma, remembered or not."[3] I recall the 45-year-old carnival roustabout who was burned over 40% of his body when his mobile home furnace exploded. His repeated dressing changes in the large tub were as painful as expected. However, he soon became unusually fearful and tremulous whenever I entered the room, but not when the nurses or the more junior members of the surgical team approached him. His exaggerated submissiveness and fear toward me apparently had some hidden explanation.

One Saturday morning I put my feet up to have a more leisurely conversation with him. Steering the conversation from his immediate family to his childhood, I asked as casually as I could

---

[2] Muller H: *The Uses of the Past.* New York, Oxford University Press, 1975, p. 34.

[3] Terr L: *Unchained Memories: True Stories of Traumatic Memories, Lost and Found.* New York, Basic Books, 1994, p. xiii.

about his father. The tears broke quickly. This paragon of machismo melted into the sad child he really was, as he poured out a story of physical beatings and abuse that continued to torture him long after he had escaped the blows by running away from home to join the circus. Being placed in a submissive and powerless role again by a man who inflicted pain brought back the original emotions and the behavior he had spent the rest of his life trying to expunge through bravado.

There was the woman in her fifties with terrible bedsores who clutched her teddy bear to her cheek and sobbed bitterly whenever we discussed plans for her treatment. As I knew she had successfully raised a large family before a mishap had taken away the feeling and use of her legs, I directed our conversation toward illnesses she might have had as a child. I learned between her sobs that she had burned her feet severely while walking barefoot through a dump at the age of 8. She had been unable to find a way out of the smoldering embers left by a rubbish fire. There followed weeks of painful treatment in the hospital at that time. Now, once more she became the same 8-year-old she had been nearly five decades earlier.

I remember the successful middle-aged businesswoman whom I found sobbing uncontrollably in the induction room before her left wrist was to undergo carpal tunnel release. My preoperative probings surprisingly failed to uncover any significant prior experience with surgeons or other physicians during childhood. Despite high doses of sedatives and successful local anesthesia, the procedure was difficult because of the shaking of her hand and body. At the time of suture removal I discovered, with a bit of probing, that while she had not undergone a surgical operation herself in childhood, she had experienced a related emotional trauma. On several occasions at age nine she had watched her older sister slash her own wrists. The tears flowed as this patient shared her horrifying memories of the blood gushing from her sister's wrists to spatter crimson patterns on the white tiles of the bathroom. The bitterness of the sordid physical and emotional abuse she had suffered at the hands of this disturbed and sadistic sibling was released from within when she was forced to confront a surgical incision into her own wrist.

The worst of all for me has always been the suffering of burned children. It is impossible not to inflict repeated pain during the necessary dressing changes on their tender raw surfaces. Their emotional reactions are always heartbreaking to me, even after all my years in intensive care units. Despite the explanations and the diversions, the pain administered by an adult is always perceived as punishment. I know that by the time they leave the hospital, their emotional lives will be as indelibly scarred as their hands and faces. I am aware that their future behavior may be driven in new and unpredictable directions by the painful stresses of their treatment. Their lives may have been extended by the treatment, but in exchange for an emotional mortgage with lifetime payments because of what I had done.

Several years ago Dartmouth Medical School Dean James Strickler mentioned to me in casual table conversation that Dr. Nathan Smith, the founder of the school, had once performed a surgical operation on the leg of Joseph Smith, the founder of the Mormon tradition. Dr. Strickler was proud of Dartmouth's early medical excellence and added that Dr. Leroy Wirthlin had carefully researched and published the story.[4] I implored Dr. Strickler to send me a photocopy of Wirthlin's article.

Having been raised in more than casual association with the Reorganized Church of Jesus Christ of Latter Day Saints, the notion of a connection between my mystical childhood world and my current profession was intriguing. The Reorganized Church, for those unfamiliar with the distinction, carries no formal affiliation with the much larger and more familiar body in Utah. It was formed instead in the Midwest under the leadership of Joseph Smith III, the Mormon prophet's son, after the westward departure of the main body under Brigham Young. My mother's family had been involved in the organization to varying degrees, and I was to find out much later (and only as I was completing work on this book) that my great-great-great-aunt had married this Joseph Smith III.

---

[4] Wirthlin LS: "Nathan Smith (1762–1828), Surgical Consultant to Joseph Smith." *BYU Studies* 17:319–337, 1977.

But if I read Wirthlin's narrative that first time through the eyes of the enchanted world of my youth, I shortly reread it with the hardened eyes of a surgeon who performs just such operations on young children. My own medical school studies in psychiatry at Harvard Medical School under Drs. John Nemiah and Frank Ervin had emphasized the importance of avoiding, if possible, those critical early to middle childhood years in the performance of circumcision, or any other elective operation for that matter, because of boys' greatest fears at that age.

This time the recognition was instantaneous. A cluster of three obscenely painful operations on the lower extremity of a 7-year-old boy without anesthesia could hardly have been experienced other than as a horrible emotional trauma with a worst case of psychological overtones. (Peter would have required no second reading.)

I soon began to ask myself what adult behavioral patterns might be expected in such an individual whose brutal childhood trauma held themes of dismemberment, punishment, and worse. Would there be allusions to this incident in his writings? in his religious rituals? What about polygamy? Was Joseph himself enmeshed in some of the plural marriage practices associated with the Mormon movement? The Reorganized Church had always vehemently denied this, but I had heard whisperings that he was more than a casual participant. Having had little to no contact with the organization for a quarter century, I was too far removed to pursue the story. Furthermore, with a busy clinical practice in two hospitals, an active research laboratory, a growing young family, and a number of other interests, this intriguing subject would have to be put off for a time.

It was four years later that the invitation came from a nearby society of plastic surgeons to address a quarterly meeting. Ordinarily there would have been a tray of slides summarizing a current laboratory or clinical topic of interest for such an occasion, but I was somehow "between projects" for the first time in my career. As my major operation for the day had been unexpectedly cancelled the morning I opened the invitation, I suddenly had several hours of precious leisure on my hands. Recalling the Wirthlin article, I walked the block-and-a-half to Dartmouth's

Baker Library to explore the matter further, in anticipation of a short and pensive after-dinner talk. I quickly discovered that trying to investigate a little bit of Mormon history is like being a little bit pregnant. I was hooked.

The story that soon began to emerge from authoritative sources concerning the grandiose behavior of Joseph Smith, Jr. was more than a little disturbing. But, I asked myself, did it automatically follow that if this quixotic man were not divine, was he therefore a willful fraud, a vicious impostor, or a promiscuous lothario? Was there another way to interpret Joseph Smith's behavior that was both internally consistent and compatible with what is known from studies of human behavior?

My hypothesis concerning Wirthlin's article suggested there might indeed be another interpretation to consider. I meekly presented some of my fragmentary thoughts to Dr. Bernard Bergen of Dartmouth's Department of Sociology. The idea of a book grew out of the meeting. For Dr. Bergen saw instantly—it seemed to me as quickly as Peter with the cook—the full scope of psychopathological patterns in the story that I had but glimpsed. He suggested to me a sizable bibliography to refresh and organize my understanding of psychoanalytic thought. My chairman, Dr. Robert Crichlow, graciously agreed to a three-month sabbatical leave in order that I might initiate the project.

But it was not until the "final" draft was completed some two or three years later that I was introduced to a far more important source than the Freudians, one that demanded that I rethink and rewrite major portions of the book. I refer to the sensitive writings of Dr. Lenore Terr, the child psychiatrist of San Francisco whose original contributions on the long-term effects of childhood trauma have brought the entire field to a new focus of understanding.[5] Terr's work and that of Dr. Leonard Shengold[6] and

---

[5] See Terr L: *Too Scared to Cry: Psychic Trauma in Childhood.* New York, Harper & Row, 1990; Terr L: *Unchained Memories: True Stories of Traumatic Memories, Lost and Found.* New York, Basic Books, 1994.

[6] Shengold L: *Soul Murder: The Effects of Childhood Abuse and Deprivation.* New York, Ballantine, 1989.

others demonstrated to me how the behavior of Joseph Smith, Jr. shared so many common features with that of others who have experienced similar humiliating and painful experiences as small children. Again, as Terr writes, "A whole life can be shaped by an old trauma, remembered or not."

And in the closing of one last circle, I unexpectedly encountered Dr. John Nemiah, my Harvard psychiatry professor of a quarter century past, at an oral presentation of my thesis. With gentle enthusiasm and warm tea he kindly helped to round out my understanding of the role of dissociation in psychopathology and how this seems to have played a role in Joseph Smith's behavior. I am grateful that in returning to his own roots in Hanover, New Hampshire, Dr. Nemiah helped me to comprehend my own.

I have come to agree with Wirthlin's conclusion that Nathan Smith was a critical player in the founding of the Mormon movement. Had there been no Nathan Smith there would have been no Mormon religion. Dr. Smith, who founded three medical schools in addition to my own, was one of a handful of great pioneers in American medicine. But it is arguable that his impact on the fabric of American life has been greater through a cluster of forgettable operations on a small boy than through the combined output of all of his medical schools. Wirthlin and I may disagree on why this is so, but not on the necessity of Nathan Smith's participation. And it is also this critical fact that has become a kind of nagging personal burden as I realize what enormous consequences can result whenever I, myself, pick up a scalpel to operate on a small child.

Perhaps my greatest surprise in studying Joseph Smith, Jr.'s life, however, came in working backward from a puzzling section of his *The Book of Mormon.* A clue lurking there opened up a line of investigation that led me to understand that the childhood operations were only half the story. The second critical event was the impact on 17-year-old Joseph of the death of his older brother Alvin. The pain of this second trauma, qualitatively different from that of the first because of its bereavement nature and the age when it was experienced, became indispensable to my understanding of some of Joseph's most bizarre behavior. Only Alvin's death, impacting on a personality wounded by the earlier trauma, would permit those mystical events of Joseph's life to flow forward in all their spontaneity. I have taken the liberty of bypassing strict chronology in introducing this second trauma in favor of sharing it the way it came to me, from *The Book of Mormon* itself.

It is expected that many readers of this book will have little to no knowledge of Mormon history and that others will know little of psychoanalytic studies. I have, therefore, tried to provide some introductory material in both disciplines. In so doing, I suspect that cognoscenti in both disciplines may find the "primer" material to be simplistic and less formally presented than would be the case in the respective professional literature of each. In the case of disputed historical events, I have tried to draw conclusions from the weight of the evidence available in the published record.

But if I found the *historical* record of my subject to be bipolar (between the divine and skeptical camps), I had no premonition whatever of the bipolar reception my work would invoke between the two disciplines themselves. Historians, in general, seemed to find my thesis improbable and full of unsupported speculation (although the earlier drafts were indeed hopelessly Freudian). Psychiatrists, on the other hand, felt that I had *insufficiently* explored many of the roads I had traveled. The nature of evidence, I found, separates us one from another as strongly as religious creed. Or, perhaps, it is merely a battle between right and left brains.

It is not imagined that this book will provide answers to all of the lingering questions surrounding the unusual life of Joseph Smith, Jr. It touches on only a few of them. The book is, rather, intended to be an addition to the ongoing dialogue about his behavior. It is hoped that it may provide some insights to further an understanding of this unique man, whose creative genius and leadership talents have, if anything, been underestimated. The book must not be read as a commentary on any institution or individual other than Joseph Smith, Jr. It is not about religion, literature, sociology, law, or even history. It is about one man—his experiences, his stresses, and the behavior that flowed therefrom. If the book seems to be peculiarly oriented toward the psychoanalytic understanding of human behavior, it is because many of the facts of the story seem to present themselves in such fashion.

It is my thesis that Joseph Smith's childhood operations and the events surrounding his brother's death had a dramatic impact on Joseph's adult behavior, playing a major role in making him different from other men. In making this case, it will be necessary to explore what is known of the impact emotional traumas and surgical operations have on the fantasies of children and on the sorts of lasting symptoms those fantasies can produce. Joseph Smith's actual operations will be viewed from this author's vantage point as a practicing surgeon. The events leading up to the writing of *The Book of Mormon* will be reexamined. In the analysis of the literary content of *The Book of Mormon* will be found repetitive allusions to the themes of the childhood operations as well as important clues to Joseph's feelings concerning his brother's untimely death. And a closer focus on this second tragic event will point toward a further understanding of Joseph's most peculiar behavior. Joseph Smith's sexuality will be reexamined in light of his early trauma, as will those rituals and metaphors that punctuated his life. The focus throughout will be on understanding his behavior in the light of contemporary understanding of children's and adolescents' reactions to events of horror.

The case I present is not predicated on the discovery (with one minor exception) of new documents or other archival information. It does not require rewriting the historical record, but merely looking at it from a fresh perspective. This perspective, I will state at the outset, has nothing to do with miracles, faith, or angels. But the question cannot be avoided concerning the extent to which some of the adult symptoms arising out of his personal horrors may now be recognized as permanent effigies in the scripture and ritual of the church he founded.

During the course of my studies, I have developed great respect for the religious creativity of Joseph Smith, Jr. His prolific contributions have been expressed in some of the most vivid imagery in the language. He was deeply preoccupied with matters of guilt, bereavement, punishment, shame, redemption, and his relationship with superiors.

Psychiatric and religious disciplines are in substantial agreement that guilt and the need to expunge it are fundamental dimensions of human existence. The two also agree on the primacy of the authoritarian relationship between child and "Father." The special privilege of studying the life of Joseph Smith, Jr. in this context has been to observe the interweaving of these two views of human existence in one man, who seems to have created a unique religious cosmology out of his own personal agonies and inner struggles. To discover a few of the highly personal origins of his guilt, to fathom some of the complexity of his view of his own father, and to try to trace how these were forged into a superstructure of powerful religious meaning that has moved millions—these have been the aims of this book.

Religion is a part of human existence precisely because of the mystery of that very existence and the need to make some meaningful sense of it. But the fact that religious themes may be dialectically reduced to projections of early parental relationships, childhood sexuality, and the confrontation with death cannot take away the impact that these themes have through their universal appeal. This quest Joseph Smith, Jr. pursued as well as Moses, and there was nothing fraudulent about his metaphorical expression of the human condition as he experienced it.

In addition to those helpful individuals I have already identified, I wish to express my gratitude to several selfless individuals whose many hours of service have contributed to this book. They include my brother Tom Morain, Ph.D., and William Russell, M.Div., J.D., without whose personal encouragement and knowledge of Mormon history I could not have completed the project. I wish to thank the many patient members of the behavioral science community who invested their knowledge in my efforts, including, especially, Norman Bernstein, M.D., Charles Solow, M.D., and Steven Gleckler, M.D. I received careful assistance from Kenneth Cramer and Philip Cronenwett in the Special Collections Division of Dartmouth's Baker Library and from Patsy Carter in the Interlibrary Loan Division. I offer special thanks to Mary Schruben, Cathy Coffin, Alice Witterschein, Alicia Green, Stephanie Hampton, Kay Mussell, and Nardi Reeder Campion, whose excellent editorial work contributed immensely to the book's completion.

The Prophet

*J*oseph Smith, Jr. was no ordinary frontier preacher. He had so inspired his thousands of followers that they would deed all their possessions to his care, travel across the ocean to tell his story, and suffer unspeakable hardship to stay by his side. He had a direct and simple style that was not lost in the most soaring metaphor of his oratory. When he delivered a revelation from God, it was unforgettable. As one witness described it:

> At once his countenance changed [and] he stood mute. Those who looked at him that day said there was a search light within him, over every part of his body. I never saw anything like it on earth. I could not take my eyes off him. He got so white that anyone who saw him would have thought he was transparent. (1)

And he carried an unparalleled measure of self-assuredness that would stand as a limitless fountain of strength to his followers and a most maddening source of resentment to his enemies.

But it was neither his manner nor the allegiance of his followers that inspired vicious assaults on his being. He had claimed to
have written a second Bible. He had announced himself to be
a prophet—God's voice on earth. He had installed himself as
lieutenant-general and commander of his own army. He would
run for president of the United States against Martin Van Buren.
He would proclaim himself King of the Kingdom of God. And he
had brazenly violated the most basic sexual taboos of the society
in which he lived. His grandiose behavior appeared to his detractors to threaten the very social fabric of American life. There
seemed to be no explanation for his behavior other than that of an
imposturous charlatan or a vainglorius madman—unless he was
really who he and his followers said he was.

It is entirely possible that Joseph Smith, Jr. was a charlatan. It
is possible that he was who he said he was. It is possible he was
both. But there may be one more possibility: that he was a dynamic, creative, and charismatic leader who was driven by powerful inner forces that neither he nor those around him could
understand or control. Could such a view reconcile those contra-
dictions and grandiose aberrations in behavior that characterized
his persona—what Mormon historian Jan Shipps has called the
"prophet puzzle"?

The Church of Jesus Christ of Latter-day Saints came to be
an extension of Joseph Smith, Jr. He had claimed to have had
a visitation at the age of fourteen from two angels who told him
that he must join none of the existing churches. An angel had
returned when he was eighteen to provide instructions on finding a book of gold plates buried in a hillside near his home in
upstate New York. This book, which he titled *The Book of Mormon,* once "translated" from its ancient language with the help
of some special stones, was alleged to be a history of the American Indians from their Hebraic origins, chronicling a visit by
Jesus Christ to these Indians in ancient times. The book conveyed an evangelical message to inform the Indians of their sacred ancestry and to bring the "gentiles" to an understanding of
its message.

With publication of *The Book of Mormon,* Joseph declared
himself to be a latter-day prophet of God and founded his church.

Baptizing dozens and ordaining most adult male members into the church's priesthood, he directed the activities of the tiny but growing cult with numerous divine prophecies. Once these pronouncements had become collated into a growing volume, the *Doctrine and Covenants,* the church counted three sacred books whereas traditional Christian churches claimed only the Bible.

Shortly after the conversion of Sidney Rigdon, a prominent Campbellite preacher from the frontier, Joseph uprooted the small body of fewer than a hundred from New York State in a move to Kirtland, Ohio. Here the organization assumed the economic structure of a communal society, with its members granting ownership of all private property to the church in much the same fashion as many other experimental societies in the America of the 1830s and 1840s.

But when Joseph decided that Kirtland would not be the New Jerusalem, he set out for the frontier and established the site for his temple in Independence, Missouri, overlooking the Missouri River at the origin of the Santa Fe Trail. By, in fact, dividing his church into two sadly undercapitalized groups hundreds of miles apart, however, even Joseph's powerful charisma could ordain neither security nor prosperity in either.

While the Kirtland group was erecting a grand temple, the Missouri Mormons were enduring some of the worst religious persecution in American history. Caught in the eddies of various social and political crosscurrents on the rough frontier, many Mormon settlers found themselves assaulted and driven from their homes. In response, Joseph marched an army of 200 men from Kirtland to western Missouri in 1834. However, on finding his followers badly outnumbered, he capitulated to the angry non-Mormon majority and withdrew to Kirtland in disgrace, leaving his New Jerusalem followers in disarray.

Despite this humiliating failure in Missouri, Joseph's group in Kirtland grew apace and completed their temple. The success bought their prophet a few years of valuable reflection to refine his message and help his church grow in complexity as well as in number. Establishing an elaborate structure of priesthood levels, Joseph yet vested ultimate authority in himself and his closest advisors. He initiated new rites of washing and purification to be performed in his temple and brought his followers to religious ecstasy at its dedication ceremonies.

But the increasing financial indebtedness of the church and its prophet would not permit the harmony to continue. With hyperinflation of land values and wild speculation on many financial fronts, Joseph founded a bank upon a grossly exaggerated capital base. Though a brief sense of prosperity would follow the issuance of the bank's paper notes, the quick collapse of the institution brought ruin and schism to the church and with it, Joseph's ignominious nocturnal flight from the city in January 1838.

His arrival in western Missouri was not unlike the return of the Prodigal Son. With the rapid influx of converts from England and elsewhere, the enthusiastic Mormon colony was expanding while simultaneously increasing the loathing of its neighbors. Joseph organized a secret army of defense and infused it with the same religious sense of mission that had characterized his temple-building. After some barbaric skirmishes by both sides, the full weight of the Missouri militia finally besieged Joseph's fortified community and extracted a harsh surrender. The prophet and a small group of confidants were taken off to jail in Liberty, Missouri, as the militia plundered the town. Joseph's skillful lieutenant Brigham Young led the banished Mormons back across the Mississippi to Illinois, where Joseph, remarkably spared execution, escaped and joined them some months later.

There, in 1839, Joseph founded the city of Nauvoo and built it from an encampment on a bend in the river to the largest city in Illinois in a scant half-decade. There, despite continuing indebtedness, he organized and administered the political and financial fortunes of his community even as he drilled a great army to defend it. There in parallel fashion, he elaborated his theology to a flowering superstructure of rite and ceremony in the mammoth rising temple that he would never live to see completed. And there he gained sufficient political influence that the courts of Illinois would protect him from extradition to Missouri.

But it was at Nauvoo, as will be discussed in Chapter 7, that Joseph could not escape from his own disillusioned disciples who would discover secrets he could no longer keep hidden. Joseph Smith, Jr. had built a society that so reflected his own internal conflicts that broad disclosure of the elements of that conflict would bring about his own destruction and tear at the fabric of that society itself. That conflict is the subject of this book.

Note

1. Lightner MER: "Remarks." Given at Brigham Young University, April 14, 1905. Typescript BYU, LDS Historical Department, Salt Lake City. See also Newell LK, Avery VT: *Mormon Enigma: Emma Hale Smith.* Garden City, NY, Doubleday and Co., 1984, p. 31.

Chapter Two

Bloodshed

Unfortunately, only the barest external framework of circumstances is known of the childhood of Joseph Smith, Jr. His family lived at the
fringe of agricultural subsistence within a few
miles of the upper Connecticut River in Vermont
and New Hampshire until Joseph was ten years
old. There his character was formed. His experiences with his parents, his siblings, and a few
other individuals during that period in his life
would firmly establish his personality. Any and all
subsequent experiences would occur against that
structure of personality, complete with a defined
sense of self and a deeply embedded set of psychological tools for dealing with the stresses of
the world around him. No subsequent event
could have engendered even a small fraction of
the impact on his behavior and character that was
induced by those events occurring prior to his departure from New England.

Although a great deal can be inferred from the
circumstances of the family's activities, only a single incident is known of Joseph Smith's own life
before the age of ten. In fact, his mother, who late

in life labored to relate her son's history, lamented that "as nothing occurred during his early life, except those trivial circumstances which are common to that state of human existence, I pass
them in silence" (1). One might expect her memory to be much
keener for the early-life experiences of Alvin, her first-born, or
Lucy, her youngest. The fourth of nine children (third of six sons)
can be expected neither to have remained very prominent in his
mother's memory nor to have been the focus of much of her dis-
tracted attention during his early life. She has said as much.

Joseph's mother and father were from respectable, but hardly
wealthy, New England lineages. But both sets of grandparents had
already experienced more satisfactory financial and social fortunes than Joseph, Sr. and Lucy Mack Smith would ever achieve
during their own twenty years in the region. One can safely sur-
mise that the couple must have felt some degree of humiliation
when their several serial efforts at earning a livelihood failed to
gain either financial comfort or social station. Both families enjoyed generally good health except for Lucy's father, Solomon
Mack, who suffered from epilepsy, presumably as a sequela of
a head injury from a fall off a horse. Most family members would
likely have witnessed the seizures or been given vivid descriptions
of them.

The couple first farmed the rocky soil near Tunbridge, Vermont, for six years and then set up a shop in town. Joseph, Sr.
soon invested both his wife's dowry and all his own money in
a speculative venture on a shipment of ginseng root, losing it all
either because the market was glutted or through a swindle. With
an accumulation of bad debts, the farm was sold, and the family, in
penury with three children, relocated to nearby Royalton. A few
months later they moved a few miles east to Sharon, Vermont,
where they rented a small portion of Lucy's father's farm and
where Joseph, Sr. added a bit to the meager income by teaching
school during the winter. At this point in the family's odyssey of
indigence, on December 23, 1805, Joseph, Jr. was born.

It may be assumed that the parents' aspirations for this extra
mouth to feed would not likely have been as ambitious as those
for Alvin, born eight years before, or Hyrum, born two years after
Alvin, when there had still existed a handsome four-figure dowry

and a farm to which the family had title. (One could also suspect that some resentment might have surfaced on Lucy's part when the dowry had had to disappear into the settling of the debts after the abortive ginseng venture.) The family of six (Sophronia had been born two-and-a-half years before Joseph) soon returned to Tunbridge, where Samuel was born two-and-a-half years after Joseph. From there they relocated to Royalton where Ephraim was born two years after Samuel (but died within two weeks), and where William was born a year later. The family of eight shortly moved across the Connecticut River to a frame house near the Mascoma River in Lebanon (now West Lebanon), New Hampshire, where Caroline was born the following year. Two more children, Don Carlos and Lucy, would come later. Joseph was six and a half when he found himself the fourth child of seven, including two older and two younger brothers. It is small wonder his mother little remembered his childhood.

There is fortunately an abundance of information concerning one particular family preoccupation—a reverence for supernatural phenomena. Some manifestations of this were evident during Joseph, Jr.'s formative period in New England. As the vast body of evidence has been documented in scholarly detail by D. Michael Quinn, I acknowledge my debt to his book *Early Mormonism and the Magic World View* (2). Joseph, Sr.'s great-grandfather and another relative had testified against the Salem witches in 1692. A neighbor of the Smith family had recalled, "This Joseph Smith, Senior, we soon learned, from his own lips, was a firm believer in witchcraft and other supernatural things; and had brought up his family in the same belief" (3). Joseph, Sr. also had related to his brother Jesse that his own belief in magic was "a golden calf [which had] brought me out of the land of Vermont."

Much of Joseph, Sr.'s practice of magic centered around his use of the divining rod. There are numerous independent reports substantiating his use of this talisman in Vermont. The rod was used to find water, to find treasure, and to reveal unknown information. According to widespread tradition of the time, the successful use of the divining rod was a "godly gift." In practice, the rod was held immobile pointing forward in the hands. When the rod was to reveal something, it began to move about, to point upward, or to point downward to locate the object. Accounts are contradictory concerning Joseph, Sr.'s participation in the odd "Wood Scrape" affair in 1802 when a group of rodsmen apocalyptically claimed the date they would inherit the region around Middletown, Vermont. But he would certainly have been a devout believer and fellow traveler in the cause. Furthermore, it is certain that he had maintained considerable affiliation with many of this loose fraternity of occultists, both before and after leaving New England.

There is substantial documentation of other family immersion in occult practices. In the first draft of Lucy Smith's history of her son, she refers to the family's "trying to win the [F]aculty of Abrac, drawing Magic circles or sooth saying." (The Faculty of Abrac, often linked to Masonry, was an occult pursuit from which was derived the magic word "abracadabra" [4].) There is one report from a neighbor after the New England years that Lucy performed various magical divinations, including palmistry (5).

It is known that the Smith family engaged in treasure hunting and "money-digging" as early as 1820 (when Joseph was fourteen years of age), using at least some of the paraphernalia of maps, stones, and rods that characterized the practice. Whether and to what extent such activity occurred during Joseph, Jr.'s earlier childhood is not terribly important so long as it is recognized that certain nonrational beliefs were shared within his family culture from the beginning. These included the discovery power of the talisman, the "gift" required to utilize it (which his father ostensibly possessed), and the belief that the practice of magic could be used to fulfill wishes. Such beliefs can give considerable opportunity to a creative and troubled mind in its confrontation with the world's stresses.

Astrology held a particular fascination for the Smith family, and a number of artifacts originally owned by them have survived that corroborate such heavy investment. Several magic parchments were used by the Smith family, some of them fashioned after known illustrations from astrological books of the times. That such books were available to them is supported by Quinn's discovery that the bookstore in Hanover, New Hampshire, the town where Hyrum Smith had attended school during the family's residence in nearby Lebanon, had advertised two books on astrology and the occult in 1799. A magic dagger has been passed down through Hyrum Smith's family, almost certainly having belonged to Joseph, Sr., for it contains an inscription of the seal of the astrological symbol of Mars, the planet governing the year of the elder Smith's birth. This dagger is typical of those known to have been used by the Smiths and their compatriots to draw magic circles in treasure-digging ceremonies, as will be detailed in Chapter 4.

Evidence for the impact of this early occult and astrological milieu on Joseph, Jr., born in a year ruled by Jupiter, is seen in the fact that he carried in his pocket until his death a silver Jupiter medallion crafted precisely according to instructions in an 1801 book of magic. The serpent-headed cane that he carried during his adult life displayed an elaborately carved magic seal of Jupiter with the symbolic message, "Jupiter reigns over Joseph Smith." Indeed, one of Joseph, Jr.'s close acquaintances in later life stated that "the only thing the Prophet [Joseph, Jr.] believed in was astrology" (6).

Although both Joseph, Sr. and Lucy professed belief in God, organized religion appears to have played no more than a traditional role in the life of their family in New England. Joseph, Sr. appeared to follow his own father's strong antichurch attitudes. Lucy was more ambivalent, having become temporarily involved in Methodist revivals in Vermont in 1810. However, she and sons Hyrum and Samuel were active members of the Palmyra Presbyterian Church from about 1820 to 1828 (7). Both parents believed firmly, however, that dreams were revelatory, of the world both as it was and as it was to be. Dreams, like the world of magic, were felt to be among the gifts of communication that men were bequeathed from the supernatural world to deal with the uncertainties of life.

There does not appear to be much in this deprived background of poverty, multiparity, rootless displacement, and supernatural world view that would suggest that anything other than more of the same might come out of it. The frequent moves from place to place must have deprived Joseph of close, lasting friendships outside the family circle. His tiny world would in all probability have been confined by limits of circumstance and poverty to his immediate family, entrapped by all of the conflicts that his position in that family doled out to him. Great men with grandiose views of their destinies in the world have been known to emerge from such squalor, even among middle children, but not without some stimulus in addition to what Joseph's mother called "those trivial circumstances which are common to that state of human existence." So far none has become apparent.

There are some additional assumptions that may be properly made. Joseph, Jr. must have become caught up in the pecking order of sibling politics in the rivalry over scarce provisions and personal attention in the teeming Smith household. He might have harbored some jealousy, as well as awe and affection, for his older brothers Alvin and Hyrum in particular. But his social aspirations in early life should hardly have extended much further than gaining preferential favor with his parents among his several siblings.

The pivotal event in Joseph's life that seems, at least in substantial part, to have profoundly altered his personality occurred shortly after his seventh birthday. At that time he underwent a cluster of surgical operations without anesthesia and was sent away from home to recuperate. The procedures themselves were expertly performed and clinically successful. But the brutal consequences for Joseph's emerging personality appear to have resulted not only from the operations themselves but also from the lamentable fact that the circumstances of those operations were similar to the age-appropriate oedipal fantasies already lurking in the child's mind. When reality met fantasy in Joseph's bedroom, its result would be cataclysmic for his personality.

This tragic clash—occurring at age seven with Joseph's cluster of operations and subsequent separation from his family—would be the progenitor not only of a body of literary output but also of a unique cosmology. Why a surgical event should have had such a soul-wrenching impact—a catastrophic emotional trauma—is the subject of a sizable body of psychoanalytic literature that must be incorporated into the story.

Joseph's older sister, Sophronia, was the first of the Smith family to be struck by the typhoid epidemic sweeping the upper

Connecticut River valley during the winter of 1812–1813. The family's physician, Dr. Parkhurst,[1] attended her for about three months before discontinuing his care. Lucy's account of the story implies that he gave Sophronia up for lost, although financial or interpersonal factors are other possible reasons for his departure. When Sophronia's illness reached a crisis, the sum of Lucy's total affections became fixed on her oldest daughter in desperation. Sophronia survived the crisis and recovered. Although Lucy's narrative describes only a clasped-hand plea by the parents to "God in prayer and supplication," it is certain that the many other channels of appeal in the parents' rich repertoire of communications skills with supernatural powers were explored as well.[2]

Lucy must have experienced a jumble of feelings at this time. In addition to feelings of affection, such moments for parents are usually laced with guilt, in part because of a sense of failure to protect the child but also as an outgrowth of their own childhood memories of punishments when loved objects were taken away for misbehavior.

Sophronia's initial attack of typhoid fever was followed in overlapping succession by attacks in Hyrum, Alvin, and the other

---

[1] Joseph, in his later account, called him Parker, but the Lebanon town historian, Robert Leavitt, knows only of a Dr. Parkhurst at that time, whose training was that he "had read a little medicine."

[2] As an historiographic aside, the nature of the book in which Lucy's account is described must be put into perspective. It was dictated during the painful aftermath of Joseph's murder when his mother was nearly seventy years of age, and with very substantial assistance from a Mormon couple, who performed an editorial as well as transcriptional service. It had a sacred rather than a secular orientation in order to legitimize the divine claims of Joseph (and, ergo, the Smith family). The narrative was very substantially revised by the church leadership in Utah before its later release in a heavily edited version. The original manuscript, referenced in this book, was republished in 1969 by Arno Press. There is scarce allusion in Lucy's account to known historical facts related to the occult, "money-digging," or other early activities that suggest other than a humble, devout life of travail and faith in preparation for Joseph's religious mission. See the excellent historiographic discussion in Shipps J: *Mormonism: The Story of a New Religious Tradition*. Urbana, IL, University of Illinois Press, 1985, pp. 90–107.

four children. It strains the imagination to envision how Lucy's already difficult life was consumed by caring at once for several bedridden children, prostrate with high fever and diarrhea. All survived. In the face of what is known of the sanitation practices of the day, it is impossible that she and her husband would not also have contracted the disease unless perhaps their symptoms were mild because of prior exposure and immunity.

Joseph, Jr. seems to have been the only one of the children to have developed complications of the disease, and it is this bit of statistical caprice (or design, as one wishes) that forms the inciting event in this phase of American religious history. After resolution of his two-week bout with fever and prostration, Joseph remained free of symptoms until a painful abscess formed in the lymph nodes of his left armpit. The physician, called in at the earliest stages of this secondary infection, misdiagnosed the pain as a sprain, prescribed some liniment, and applied "the hot shovel," a form of warm compress.

On the second visit, made after two weeks of steadily increasing pain and progressive swelling, the diagnosis was obvious. An incision would have to be made into the abscess to drain the pus. The necessary lancet was produced and plunged into the swollen skin to release "fully a quart" of pus. There is no description of the circumstances of this minor operation, but from what is known of young boys' age-appropriate fantasies of men bearing knives, the scene may be readily imagined. The result, however—the immediate relief of the source of two weeks' pain—would have made the uncomfortable event a tolerable burden that by itself might well have been quickly forgotten. This sort of minor invasion of the body is usually borne well by any child who must suffer through the equivalent discomfiture of the removal of a splinter from a finger.

There was to be a second complication, however. The *Salmonella typhi* bacteria had already spread through his bloodstream to the upper portion of his left tibia, the shinbone, where the marrow was being replaced by a second abscess. As is the natural history of this condition, called *osteomyelitis,* the abscess expanded to involve the layer of tissue just beneath the periosteum, the nourishing membrane ensheathing the bone. This nerve-rich sheath was expanded by the growing pocket of pus, and this expansion caused pain greater than any he had ever experienced. (Indeed, it is widely reported that periosteal pain is more severe than that of any other tissue.) The intervening bone on the front surface of Joseph's tibia was deprived of its blood supply and died. Pus produced a massive swelling on the front of his leg. This most painful stage of the illness lasted a full two weeks. Any seven-year-old would have found such a noxious event to be terribly frightening and excruciating.

The two existing accounts of these events are in considerable agreement. Joseph described the period of the illness as follows:

> The doctors broke the fever, after which it settled under my shoulder. . . . When it proved to be a swelling under the arm which was opened, and discharged freely, after which the disease removed and descended into my left leg and ancle and terminated in a fever sore of the worst kind, and I endured the most acute suffering for a long time. (8)[3]

His mother related:

> As soon as the sore had discharged itself the pain left it and shot like lightning (using his own terms) down his side into the marrow of the bone of his leg and soon became very severe. My poor boy, at this, was almost in despair, and he cried out, "Oh, father! the pain is so severe, how can I bear it!" (9)

Now for a short period, perhaps one of few in his young life, Joseph Smith, Jr. appears to have been permitted the sole nurturing attention of his mother. As it had with the oldest daughter, all of the powerful mixture of maternal emotions induced by her child's illness rallied Lucy's attention now to the cause of her middle son. He was suffering and in mortal danger. But even this protective, grieving mother was not omnipotent:

---

[3] The idiosyncrasies in the spelling of Joseph Smith, Jr. and his several scribes are numerous, as the reader will note throughout the passages reproduced in this book. This will be noted especially in quotations taken from the first edition of *The Book of Mormon*. Therefore, for purposes of readability, no attempt has been made to indicate where these occur by tediously interjecting the term *sic* throughout the text.

> During this period I carried him much of the time in my
> arms in order to mitigate his suffering as much as possible;
> in consequence of which I was taken very ill myself. The
> anxiety of mind that I experienced, together with my physi-
> cal over-exertion, was too much for my constitution and my
> nature sank under it. (10)

Did Lucy contract typhoid fever herself at this time? Did she
suffer "nervous collapse" in a frenzy of sleep deprivation and frustration over her son's pain? Did she suffer depression? Might she
have been more successful in bearing the awful stress if the pain
had been Sophronia's again, or perhaps Alvin's, her firstborn?
From Joseph's vantage point, however, the admitted failure of his
mother's nurturing at this point of crisis must have been dreadful.
It is reasonable to assume that the seven-year-old perceived his
mother's actions as rejection and betrayal at best or as some form
of punishment at worst. His age-specific powerful affection for his
mother—once all but realized at the moment of his greatest physical pain—could not have been relinquished without enormous
disappointment.

His mother absent, Joseph would content himself with the
nurturing substitute of his older brother Hyrum, whose presence,
though comforting, would certainly have been second best for the
suffering child. As Lucy relates:

> Hyrum, who was rather remarkable for his tenderness and
> sympathy, now desired that he might take my place. As he was
> a good trusty boy, we let him do so, and, in order to make the
> task as easy as possible, we laid Joseph upon a low bed and
> Hyrum sat beside him, almost day and night for some consid-
> erable length of time, holding the affected part of his leg in his
> hands and pressing it between them, so that his afflicted
> brother might be enabled to endure the pain which was so ex-
> cruciating that he was scarcely able to bear it. (11)

After three weeks of agony, the parents called in "the surgeon." Why the boy should have had to suffer unattended this
long is unknown and, by today's standards, unconscionable. Perhaps relations with familiar physicians had soured. Perhaps other

"treatments" in the family's repertoire were being used. Or perhaps the thought of another knife-wielding adult male was too
overwhelming for young Joseph, who might have defiantly preferred to bear the pain that he knew rather than the fear that he
could imagine.

The second surgical event, the first on his leg, would have reinforced the anxiety of the former procedure through its repetition. In addition to strengthening the inevitable dismemberment
fantasies of the young boy, it should certainly have carried far
greater physical pain. Joseph surely offered more resistance
against the surgeon's efforts on this occasion. Physical restraint
would likely have been necessary to carry out the drainage procedure, and the resulting physical deformity should have appeared
hideous to any young boy's self-image. Lucy described the procedure as follows:

> When [the surgeon] came he made an incision of eight
> inches, on the front side of the leg, between the knee and
> ankle. This relieved the pain in a great measure, and the pa-
> tient was quite comfortable until the wound began to heal,
> when the pain became as violent as ever. (12)

One can scarcely imagine Joseph's state of fear during those
days and nights as the pain in his leg returned in ever-increasing
intensity. He knew the surgeon would certainly have to return to
slash again at the open wound whose swollen edges had become
so tender they could not bear even the gentlest touch. His mother
had "abandoned" him, he had barely slept in weeks because of the
pain (and nightmares), and the sight and smell of the oozing mess
that used to be his left leg would have repulsed any seven-year-old
into a state of panic.

The surgeon returned for a second assault on the limb. Again,
with whatever bodily restraints were required, he slashed more
deeply into Joseph's flesh, this time separating the swollen tissues
from the underlying tibial bone in a futile attempt to open the
labyrinth of pus pockets. But this too would prove insufficient, for
Joseph's infection was not focused in the soft tissues but in the
tibia itself. His mother's detachment during this phase of his ill-

ness is perhaps subtly revealed in her narrative by her lack of detail concerning her son's reactions to this operation. His conduct
should have been indelibly burned into her memory had she witnessed it.

By now Joseph's emotional health should have been as precarious as that of his left leg. It is doubtful that he would have
maintained at this time any of the normal controls on his behavior
that his family had previously come to expect. More likely, he
would have regressed to more infantile behavior, even including
loss of bladder and bowel control, with outbursts and nightmares
of the most horrible kind.[4] But the worst was yet to come.

The climactic moment soon arrived. Joseph found himself
faced with a kind of ritualistic assembly of eleven somber doctors
who had come to the house to make the final assault on his limb.
He had seen some of them before and had tried to forget. He
knew the bondage, the searing pain of the knives, the accursed
failure of his parents to protect him, the threat of dismemberment, the punishment, the loss. How could this be happening
once again? Was there no escape from this repetition of torture? As
he heard the cluster of hoofbeats out front, heard the surgeons
enter the front door and whisper with his mother, watched them
enter the room, he knew (as surely as today's burned child knows
when the stretcher arrives at his or her hospital bedside) what
would come next.

He watched his mother leave the room. If she hadn't left on
her own, she would have been obliged to leave. In traditional
Western culture, women do the nurturing until it is time for the
violence. (Midwives deliver babies, but men do the cesarean sec-
tions; women feed the chickens, but men butcher them.) It was
not her place to stay. It was his father who would help the surgeons restrain him.

Lucy knew that, and the twelve men remaining, including her
husband, knew that—but did Joseph? Could it for him have been
the final betrayal, the final abandonment, the final confirmation

---

[4] One sees Joseph's equivalent today in the severely burned child who must
face the twice-daily agony of bloody dressing changes at the hands of
seemingly merciless adults.

of that fantasy of his age? Having tasted the sweetness of her deepest affections such a short time ago and having already experienced a limited preview of her rebuff, did he witness her departure in this ritualistic drama of his bedroom as a climactic act of betrayal?

Fear had by now certainly driven rational understanding of these terrible events from the child's mind. The repressed fears would likely have been erupting with waves of terror as fantasy and reality converged in the sleep-deprived chaos of his psyche. Something inside him—something of which he, at age seven, was but vaguely aware—must have known his father's companions could exact the ultimate punishment. His assaulted leg at some level of consciousness would become a powerful symbol for the terrible conflict of childhood fantasy that he would never resolve. Had they come to cut it off?

The instrument case was reopened. Joseph would have dreaded viewing its contents once again. The chief surgeon, Nathan Smith, always brought the complete set, for in his memoirs he had written, "When we undertake this operation, we should be provided with all the instruments named, as we cannot always forsee [*sic*] at the commencement of the operation, what instruments we shall need before it is finished" (13). Most of all, Joseph would have feared the amputation knife, that foot-long, sword-like instrument whose design had not appreciably changed in the hundreds of years since the primitive barber-surgeons. Most surgical instrument kits carried two or even three. That "sword"—its pain and its ultimate purpose—had haunted his dreams and daytime fantasies since it had been first (and for a second time) plunged into his leg. The sword would not cease occupying those fantasies, ever.

The swollen, pus-filled tissues were cleaved once again. The sensitive periosteum was stripped. The trephine was drilled and twisted into the bone. The largest chunk of dead bone was pried free with a hook. Blood poured after it. Forceps grabbed smaller chunks and forcefully dislodged them from the fresh edges of sensitive living tissue. Saws cut through the margins. The geyser of blood was stemmed with cloth packing, and then it was over. Joseph's leg would one day heal. His psyche would not.

This scenario is the most plausible one for the events that occurred that day in this author's experience in caring for many burned children and in suturing hundreds of children's lacerations in emergency rooms. The author has frequently seen small children strike their parents after being released from restraints for suture of a laceration in an emergency room. Children, expecting parents to protect them from adults who cause pain, often display anger when parents help the doctor instead.

Lucy Mack Smith, who seemed by the time of this final operation to have recovered her spirit and her empathy, narrated the following account of her presurgical conference with the Dartmouth physicians:

> . . . we deemed it wisdom to call a council of surgeons; and when they met in consultation, they decided that amputation was the only remedy.
>
> Soon after coming to this conclusion, they rode up to the door, and were invited into a room, apart from the one in which Joseph lay. They being seated, I addressed them thus: "Gentlemen, what can you do to save my boy's leg?" They answered, "We can do nothing; we have cut it open to the bone and find it so affected that we consider his leg incurable and that amputation is absolutely necessary in order to save his life."
>
> This was like a thunder bolt to me. I appealed to the principal surgeon, saying, "Dr. Stone, can you not make another trial? Can you not, by cutting around the bone, take out the diseased part, and perhaps that which is sound will heal over, and by this means you will save his leg? You will not, you must not, take off his leg, until you try once more. I will not consent to let you enter his room until you make me this promise."
>
> After consulting a short time with each other, they agreed to do as I had requested, then went to see my suffering son. One of the doctors, on approaching his bed, said, "My poor boy, we have come again." "Yes," said Joseph, "I see you have; but you have not come to take off my leg, have you, sir?" "No," replied the surgeon, "it is your mother's request

that we make one more effort and that is what we have now come for." (14)

This is indeed a very compelling account of the intuitive wisdom of a protective mother. It is also a fabrication.

The "surgeons" in this case were a group of Dartmouth medical students led by Dr. Nathan Smith, the founder of Dartmouth Medical School in Hanover, New Hampshire (and later the founder of the Yale School of Medicine, of Bowdoin Medical School, and, in part, of the University of Vermont School of Medicine). Nathan Smith had been the fifth graduate of Harvard Medical School and had studied in London and Edinburgh before starting his professorial duties at Dartmouth. He had, in fact, planned to leave Dartmouth for Yale in 1812 but delayed his move specifically because of the overwhelming professional demands of the local typhoid epidemic (15).[5]

Among Dr. Smith's valuable original contributions to the science of surgery was the limb-sparing treatment of osteomyelitis (bone infection) of the long bones. His scholarly manuscript on the subject, with a fairly accurate description of the disease process and its successful treatment by removal of dead bone, was published in his memoirs in 1831 (17). However, this account is not appreciably different from the descriptions of the disease and its treatment that were contained in the surviving class notes of

---

[5] As an aside, though both Joseph and Lucy Smith refer to a "Dr. Stone," there was no physician by that name who could have been there from what is known of the historical record. There was a first-year Dartmouth medical student in 1813 named Experience P. Storrs, from Lebanon, New Hampshire, who would leave medical school shortly to enter law. Although there could have been a misrecollection of Storrs's name, it is most unlikely he would have played any role as leader or spokesman as Lucy's account suggests. This leads to the interesting speculation that the name Stone is a kind of "Freudian slip." As will be seen in later chapters, the "stone" was to become in Joseph's life a powerful and important talisman, enabling him to perform many wondrous tasks. It is possible that the enormous power that he associated with his memory of Nathan Smith became associated in his mind with the power of his seer-stone and resulted in an unconscious misnaming of his surgeon in accordance with the attributes of his talisman. The original author of the slip, of course, could have been either Joseph or his mother (16).

several of his students at Dartmouth as early as 1812. Of the disease process itself one student transcribed:

> Necrosis, mortification or death of the bones. Subjects of this disease are generally young, oftenest boys, and attacked before the age of puberty. . . . The death of bone commences by severe pain, and inflamation [*sic*] of it, and febrile symptoms are coexistent with the pain and inflamation. A common error of the present day is that matter forms in the soft parts over the bone, and thence corrupts the bone, but not usually so. . . . The disease terminating with the death of the bone. . . . The pain in these cases is often first felt in the joint below the inflamed bone, as in the ankle if the tibia be affected. . . . A fluctuation circumscribed by hardness is easily found on the tibia. . . . This inflamitory [*sic*] affection has its seat between the periosteum and bone. In the long bones both between the external and internal periosteum and the intermediat[e] bone. Medullary substance is often destroyed. In this case there is bone between the collections of matter and circulation to it being cut off, it must die. (18)

Nathan Smith was probably alone in American medicine at this time in arguing vehemently against amputation and in favor of limited removal of the dead portion of bone. As he described in clear detail in his memoirs,

> The object, however, in every case is the same; that is to remove a piece of dead bone, which has become a foreign body as it relates to the living . . .
> The instruments which may be wanted in this operation are a probe, knife, round saw, and one or more of Heys saws, several pair of strong forceps and a pair of cutting forceps. The elevator used in trepanning the skull is also an instrument which is often required in such operations.
> When I first began to perform operations of the kind, I was under apprehension lest so much bruising and handling of the soft parts, as is sometimes necessary, to dislodge a large sequestra unfavorably situated, might be followed with bad consequences, and some of these operations have

been the most laborious and tedious, both to myself and the patient, which I have ever performed. (19)

Thus, it was *not* Lucy Smith's flash of surgical insight and persuasive power that convinced the pessimistic surgeons to do as she "had requested" in saving Joseph's leg. The passage of years and her own difficult conflict in dealing with the painful event seem to have reversed the events in her own world of fantasy.

In her distorted narrative she was not the powerless, frustrated person she most certainly had been at the critical moment of Joseph's crisis. She would instead become the power broker in the story, directing Dr. Nathan Smith and his medical students to sit down in her living room, describing the ideal operation to them, and defiantly blocking their entry into Joseph's room until they changed their inadequate notions of treatment to conform to her intuitive knowledge of surgery. She would observe triumphantly as Nathan Smith humbly explained to her son that they were going to save his leg by following his mother's orders rather than their own inclinations.

She too had suffered. In her mélange of emotion, she too could scarcely have avoided feeling a measure of guilt over the possibility that this horrible event was in some way her own punishment. Most parents do in like circumstances. And she had taken to bed at the time of her son's greatest need. Such thoughts are intolerable to a mother. The story would come out with understandable distortion as she recalled the painful event many years later.

Lucy's vivid description of the events surrounding the operation itself have a surreal spin that bestows a temperate and selfless serenity upon her son:

> The principal surgeon, after a moment's conversation, ordered cords to be brought to bind Joseph fast to a bedstead; but to this Joseph objected. The doctor, however, insisted that he must be confined, upon which Joseph said very decidedly, "No, doctor, I will not be bound, for I can bear the operation much better if I have my liberty." "Then," said Dr. Stone, "will you drink some brandy?"
>
> "No," said Joseph, "not one drop."

"Will you take some wine?" rejoined the doctor. "You must take something, or you can never endure the severe operation to which you must be subjected."

"No," exclaimed Joseph, "I will not touch one particle of liquor, neither will I be tied down; but I will tell you what I will do—I will have my father sit on the bed and hold me in his arms, and then I will do whatever is necessary in order to have the bone taken out." Looking at me, he said, "Mother, I want you to leave the room, for I know you cannot bear to see me suffer so; father can stand it, but you have carried me so much, and watched over me so long, you are almost worn out." Then looking up into my face, his eyes swimming in tears, he continued. "Now, mother, promise me that you will not stay, will you? The Lord will help me, and I shall get through with it."

To this request I consented, and getting a number of folded sheets, and laying them under his leg, I retired, going several hundred yards from the house in order to be out of hearing.

The surgeons commenced operating by boring into the bone of his leg, first on one side of the bone where it was affected, then on the other side, after which they broke it off with a pair of forceps or pincers. They thus took away large pieces of the bone. When they broke off the first piece, Joseph screamed out so loudly, that I could not forbear running to him. On my entering the room, he cried out, "Oh, mother, go back, go back; I do not want you to come in—I will try to tough it out, if you will go away."

When the third piece was taken away, I burst into the room again—and oh, my God! what a spectacle for a mother's eye! The wound torn open, the blood still gushing from it, and the bed literally covered with blood. Joseph was pale as a corpse, and large drops of sweat were rolling down his face, whilst upon every feature was depicted the utmost agony!

I was immediately forced from the room, and detained until the operation was completed; but when the act was accomplished, Joseph put upon a clean bed, the room cleared of every appearance of blood, and the instruments which were used in the operation removed, I was permitted again to enter. (20)

As a surgeon, this author can say that Lucy's description of Joseph's behavior is so atypical of a seven-year-old boy facing a surgical assault that one is tempted to dismiss the entire narrative out of hand. However, it is possible that her portrayal of Joseph as a brave victim may have had a grain of validity, but only under a very special condition. It is typical of children who suffer *repeated* bouts of terrible trauma that they may enter a kind of trance or "self-hypnosis" that protects against the emotional experience of the horror. A kind of depersonalization supervenes so that the event is experienced as though it were being viewed from the outside. Lucy's narrative suggests that this may have been Joseph's maiden voyage into "dissociation." There would be many more.

Although it cannot be known how successful Joseph's dissociation was in blotting out the pain, there is inferential evidence in the later biographical record that some measure of a struggle ensued that Lucy's departure prevented her from witnessing. Joseph, Sr. no doubt tried to help the medical students restrain his son's savage struggling out of some sense of embarrassment at his son's conduct. Any parent would have done so (and most still do). But to Joseph, any such actions on his father's part could easily have confirmed to him his father's central complicity in the act. Had his father guessed those private fantasies? Why else could he be helping to inflict such unspeakable punishment? His father and his father's "friends" were extracting their final punishment—the one he had dreaded the most and the one he "probably deserved."

Regardless, if after all the pain of his three recent operations without anesthesia, his many consecutive sleepless nights, his fear of amputation and permanent disfigurement, and his immediate prospect of suffering much greater pain than ever before—if he was indeed calm and reasonable, articulate, trusting of his mother's judgment, certain of his ability to endure the pain without withdrawing, more interested in his moral purity than in pharmacological protection from his discomfort, loving of his kind and gentle father, and far more concerned with his mother's emotional welfare than his own—then seven-year-old Joseph Smith, Jr. was at that moment not "brave" but rather "somewhere else." Like the young protagonist in Hannah Green's sensitive novel *I Never Promised You a Rose Garden* (21), who unfeelingly pushed lighted cigarettes into her arms during her own postsurgical mental illness, Joseph had found a refuge from the pain by tenaciously splitting it from consciousness. He would never have conscious memory of his final operation.

The aftermath must have doubled the hurt. As soon as Joseph could travel, his parents sent him away! Probably never having been separated from his parents and siblings before in his life, he was now to be deprived of his family's reassurance at the worst possible moment. During this time, when he could have been comforted by those whose understanding and caring he so desperately needed, he would instead be sent off with his Uncle Jesse to Salem, Massachusetts, "for the benefit of his health, hoping the sea-breezes would be of service to him" (22). The journey itself had to have been physically painful, judging from the known state of roads of the era and the rugged geography that would necessarily have been traversed from the New Hampshire's western border to the seacoast. Since the fear of dismemberment is invariably associated with the fear of abandonment in a boy's mind, this reinforcement of his conflict must have been doubly devastating. Whether his parents sent him away for *his* health or *theirs,* one might expect the effect to have been the same on this brutally traumatized boy. The absence of the familiarity and affection of his family was to be one more crashing blow that his mortally wounded psyche would have to endure. Surely a very different boy returned from Salem.

It was probably in his exile at the seashore that the fantasies began, projected from within by an unspeakable horror he could not recall. As will be seen, these included huge, violent fantasies. Fantasies of wars. Fantasies of people in chaos who escape to the seashore. Fantasies of magic swords that dismember heads and arms. Fantasies of sons overthrowing fathers, princes killing kings, righteous killing unrighteous. Fantasies of towers, trees, serpents, flaming swords, pillars, cigar-shaped boats, sickles, and "stiff-necked" people. Fantasies of evil men brought to humiliation by young heroes. Fantasies of good fathers and evil fathers, of faithful women and whores. Fantasies of good armies and bad armies pushing one another to-and-fro like battles of ants. Fantasies of betrayal. Fantasies of darkness, of magic stones that light up the darkness. Fantasies of good white people and evil black people, of good white people becoming evil black people. Fantasies of princes being "bound with cords," of "blood on garments," of maggots eating flesh. Fantasies of destroying angels with drawn swords. The fantasies would flood out of his unconscious in hundreds of repetitive dreams and nightmares, in daydreams, in random sequences, in play, in speech, and in silence. They took over the inner life of Joseph Smith, Jr. as automatic pilot takes over an aircraft. In this state he limped into his future.

Notes

1. Smith LM: *Biographical Sketches of Joseph Smith the Prophet and His Progenitors for Many Generations.* Liverpool, S. W. Richards, 1853 [reprinted New York, Arno Press, 1969], p. 73.
2. Quinn DM: *Early Mormonism and the Magic World View.* Salt Lake City, Signature Books, 1987.
3. Lapham F: Statement, 1870. Quoted in Quinn DM: *Early Mormonism and the Magic World View,* p. 28.
4. Smith L: "Preliminary Manuscript," Fragments 1–10. Salt Lake City, LDS Church Archives, p. 40. Reproduced in Vogel D (ed): *Early Mormon Documents,* Vol. 1. Salt Lake City, Signature Books, 1996, p. 285.
5. Eaton H: *The Origin of Mormonism.* 1881. See *Deseret News Church Section* [Salt Lake City], May 25, 1940, pp. 5–6; see also Quinn M: *Early Mormonism and the Magic World View,* p. 56.
6. Wyl W: *Mormon Portraits, or the Truth about Mormon Leaders from 1830–1886.* Salt Lake City, Tribune Printing & Publishing Co., 1886, p. 19. See Quinn M: *Early Mormonism and the Magic World View,* p. 58.
7. Brodie F: *No Man Knows My History: The Life of Joseph Smith, the Mormon Prophet,* 2nd Edition. New York, Alfred A. Knopf, 1989, p. 410.

8. Smith J: *Manuscript History of the Church*, Book A-1. Salt Lake City, LDS Church Historian's Office, 1838, p. 131. See also Durham RC: "Joseph Smith's Own Story of a Serious Childhood Illness." *BYU Studies* 10(Summer):480–482, 1970.

9. Smith LM: *Biographical Sketches of Joseph Smith the Prophet*, p. 62.

10. Ibid., pp. 62–63.

11. Ibid., p. 63.

12. Ibid.

13. Smith N: *Medical and Surgical Memoirs.* Edited with addenda by Smith NR. Baltimore, Wm. A. Francis, 1831, p. 119

14. Smith LM: *Biographical Sketches of Joseph Smith the Prophet*, pp. 63–64.

15. Wirthlin LS: "Nathan Smith (1762–1828): Surgical Consultant to Joseph Smith." *BYU Studies* 17:319–337, 1977.

16. See Freud S: *The Psychopathology of Everyday Life* (1901). Translated and edited by Brill AA. New York, Modern Library, 1938, pp. 35–149.

17. Smith N: *Medical and Surgical Memoirs.*

18. Farnsworth S: "Nathan Smith's class notes, Lecture 2." Dartmouth Medical School, October 20, 1812. Archives, Baker Library, Dartmouth College, Hanover, NH.

19. Smith N: *Medical and Surgical Memoirs,* pp. 118–120.

20. Smith LM: *Biographical Sketches of Joseph Smith the Prophet*, pp. 64–65.

21. Green H: *I Never Promised You a Rose Garden.* New York, Holt, Rinehart, & Winston, 1964.

22. Smith LM: *Biographical Sketches of Joseph Smith the Prophet*, p. 65.

Strategic Defenses

Much of Joseph's permanent personality structure evolved during the aftermath of his surgical operations and exile as he adjusted to his role as the family's crippled child. He would hobble about on crutches for three years until his family moved from New England. In the process, he would pluck out, by his count, an additional fourteen sequestra of dead bone from his leg before it healed. His slight limp in adult life would always be a reminder of this painful period of his childhood, and he would often carry a long, rigid cane. Emotionally he would be forever maimed by this cluster of surgical events, a portion of whose memory was unavailable but whose specter he could never expunge from the dissociated recesses of his mind.

This is not to say that his bruised psyche did not try, for there is a kind of trap hidden for the reader in Lucy Smith's vivid narrative of her son's final operation. The trap is in the assumption that if she has such detailed visual memories of the event that Joseph must also. Joseph's own recollections are as follows:

> . . . the disease removed and descended into my left leg and
> ancle and terminated in a fever sore of the worst kind, and
> I endured the most acute suffering for a long time under the
> care of Drs. Smith, Stone and Perkins, of Hanover. At one
> time eleven Doctors came from Dartmouth Medical College,
> at Hanover, New Hampshire, for the purpose of amputation,
> but, young as I was, I utterly refused to give my assent to the
> operation, but consented to their Trying an experiment by
> removing a large portion of the bone from my left leg, which
> they did, and fourteen additional pieces of bone afterwards
> worked out before my leg healed, during which time I was
> reduced so very low that my mother could carry me with
> ease. (1)

There is unmistakable sadness and pain in this narrative but not
even a trace of the episode of violence that so horrified Lucy. The
difference is striking. It is important to ask why.

As suggested previously, Joseph likely did not remember the
horror of the final operation. Or, at least, he did not remember it
as Lucy's mind did. The experience did not likely exist in what is
called conscious memory. In other words, Joseph seems to have
demonstrated *amnesia* for the events of at least the final operation.

Amnesia is not so much a loss of memory as a separation of
a memory into a different realm of the mind, where it becomes
"dissociated" from conscious thought and unavailable to be
"thought about." But the repression of such memories from the
conscious sphere is never complete. The memories, instead, tend
to burst out at times of stress that are in some way reminiscent of
the original event. The forgotten memories also harbor an explosive energy that ensures that their reappearance will be loaded
with emotion. It is also worth noting Lenore Terr's observation
that home is the most common setting out of which abuse and violence will cause children to dissociate (2). In analyzing Joseph
Smith's adult behavior, his writings, and his personality, patterns
must therefore be recognized that represent the brutal trauma he
suffered—patterns mimicking the surgical tools, their anatomic
target, the perpetrators, and the underlying theme of fantasy that
was age-appropriate for Joseph when the operations occurred.

In this sense, dissociation may be regarded as an important defense of Joseph's mind. It allowed his mind to "flee" what his body was experiencing. The magnitude of the shock of the trauma was so great and the state of mind it produced so different from ordinary waking life that it became impossible to integrate the event with normal experience. This discontinuity, in turn, caused the horrific event to be lost to conscious memory or to be remembered only as a dream or as something unreal or vague. The memory, instead, was stored in the mind like a locked file in a computer, with, as it were, a password or key required to gain access. The password, in turn, would be some experience—some situation or encounter—that was in some way reminiscent of the circumstances of the trauma.

Joseph Smith, Jr. demonstrated a range of symptoms all his life that suggest he had a dissociated memory of at least part of the horrors of his childhood operations hiding in amnesia in his mind. He was aware of having had a sore leg. He was aware of having been under the care of doctors, and he was aware that at least one operation had been performed. He was aware of his family's concern. He was aware of his exile at the seashore. But it is most doubtful that he retained any conscious memory of that final operation itself—the restraints, the complicitous role of his father, the "abandonment" by his mother, the twelve somber assailants, the childhood fantasy whose theme the operations dramatized, and the fearsome amputation knife. All of these were evidently forced into amnesia because they were simply too horrible to absorb. They would never return to Joseph's conscious memory. But the lurking dissociated memory would become a dominant force in what made him different from other men.

A distinction might be made between two different manifestations of dissociation, as they are both seen in contemporary clinical situations as well as in Joseph's own life. The first was involuntary and served as a defense against pain. This manifestation was presumably a pattern that had been "learned," at least in part, through the repetitive nature of his childhood operations. Through this process he was dissociated from the stressful reality of the present. But Joseph seems also to have trained himself to use his capacity for dissociation at will in a kind of volitional self-hypnosis. This trancelike state evidently became a principal source of his creativity, presumably because of the horrible richness of content lurking in its dissociated sphere. Willing himself to tap into it was Joseph's key to distinction among men. And the plausible belief that this sphere existed *above* rather than *within* has made its impact on history.

It was as true with Joseph as with many other children who undergo psychic trauma—and by that is meant a horrible event or events that the children are utterly helpless to prevent or alter—that they will always unconsciously "choose" guilt in preference to shame as they attempt to explain the event to themselves. That is, children will fabricate a made-up reason for a tragedy and feel guilty about that fabrication in preference to feeling the humiliation of being victimized by the world's randomness. As Terr points out,

> Shame comes from public exposure of one's own vulnerability. Guilt, on the other hand, is private. It follows from a sense of failing to measure up to private, internal standards. When others "know" that you once were helpless, you tend to feel ashamed. *They* know. If, on the other hand, you feel you caused your own problems, you cease feeling so vulnerable and blame yourself, instead, for the shape of events. *You* know. But you are the only one. (3)

There is substantial biographical evidence that Joseph Smith, Jr. operated throughout his life on this fundamental psychodynamic. The guilt he experienced in his trauma appears, in part, to have flowed out of the oedipal fantasy that was appropriate for his age at the time. As a consequence, Joseph's adult sexuality seems to have been characterized by an inability to segregate eroticism from the imminent threat of violent punishment. In addition, he would be confined to a bipolar world of black and white, peopled by those who threatened and those who did not, forever barred from the myriad subtleties of color through which life should normally derive its richness.

This is not to say that Joseph's psychic life was dull—much the contrary. As is now known of the behavior of traumatized children, Joseph quite likely filled his leisurely moments with visualizations of the event in many forms. His trauma probably became reenacted in play and in dreams through endless visual images. Indeed, his mother reported that during his teen years he would regale his family with vivid stories of imaginary characters for hours as the hidden memory propelled his creative instincts (4). But the themes remained narrow—themes of helplessness, of ugly and unanticipated death in huge numbers, of betrayal, of the randomness of the world, of trauma, of swords, of shame, of dismemberment, of blood on garments, and of evil-father representations. These themes never changed. And the play didn't stop around age twelve, as typically is the case with the majority of children, but continued into adulthood. That is the way it is with traumatized children. The play became contagious and drew others into its orbit. That feature, too, is eerily common in the games of traumatized children. And of course, along with many other writers, Joseph expressed his trauma in literary fashion. In particular, says Shengold, "Artistic creativity involves a change from passive suffering of childhood traumatic experiences to active manipulation and re-creation of these experiences" (5). Or, as Elizabeth Waites describes it, "Human beings . . . do not merely suffer or inflict suffering. They interpret suffering, invent myths to explain it, and prescribe rituals to control it" (6).[1]

---

[1] There is a contemporary parallel to this form of literary creativity in the person of Stephen King, whose prolific outpouring of tales of horror has frightened and captivated millions. As Terr has described in her study of this unusual author, King experienced his own episode of childhood horror at the age of four. It seems that young Stephen had been playing along the railroad tracks with his best friend. He wandered home "as white as a ghost" in a kind of mute trance and did not speak for the rest of the day. His friend was found to have been struck by a train and was so mutilated that the dismembered pieces of his body were picked up in a wicker basket. It is likely that the author-to-be directly observed the horrible event, but no one knows. King has never been able to recall what he saw that afternoon. What is known is that he began to write hideous stories of graphic horror at the age of seven and has never stopped. As Terr states, "As a boy, King began writing because he needed to. . . . A sufferer—always—of terrible dreams and insomnia, he conveyed his nightmares to people through his writing" (7). And if anyone doubts the role of the amnestic event in driving the author's creativity, it is only necessary to view

At times in Joseph's dissociated "world apart," his fantasies seemed to flood over him, propelling him into a trancelike state. He shared that trait with others who have suffered trauma in childhood, with vivid hallucinations often accompanying these trances. Such episodes are typically difficult for onlookers to describe, but there is no mistaking their occurrence. During these dissociated states of the mind, painful memories characteristically are visualized in vivid and detailed scenes. In John Nemiah's words, these persons

> are out of contact with their environment, appear preoccupied with a private world, and, if their eyes are open, are seen to be staring into space. They may appear emotionally upset, speak excitedly in words and sentences that are frequently hard to understand, or engage in a pattern of seemingly meaningful activities that is repeated every time an episode occurs. It can often be determined that their behavior represents the external manifestations of the inner, hallucinatory reexperiencing of a traumatic event. (8)

This characterization opens new insight into Mary Elizabeth Rollins Lightner's description of Joseph's inspired moments, already quoted in Chapter 1:

> At once his countenance changed [and] he stood mute . . . there was a search light within him, over every part of his body. I never saw anything like it on earth. . . . He got so white that anyone who saw him would have thought he was transparent. (9)

This recounting is matched by a description of Joseph's 1834 exhortation to a congregation in Pontiac, Michigan:

> His countanance seemed to me to assume a heavenly whit[e]ness and his voice was so peirseing and forcible for

---

the "train trestle" scene in the movie *Stand by Me* to experience something of what King undoubtedly saw but cannot remember. Joseph Smith, Jr. shared with Stephen King that momentary bit of childhood history, and his own horror was no less dreadful. Both were driven to express the pain throughout their lives, each in a uniquely recognizable pattern of disguise.

my part it so impressed me as to become indellibly im-
printed on my mind. (10)

Terr describes such dissociated states as "a loss of color and later
with a glassy-eyed stare" (11).

Joseph would come to share an additional trait in common
with other victims of childhood trauma suffering with dissociative
symptoms: the belief that he was "psychic," or had paranormal
gifts of clairvoyance. Dreams were, after all, a method of predict-
ing the future in the Smith family's cosmology. Terr's studies with
traumatized children typically showed this self-perception to be
an outgrowth of repetitive dreaming and the skewing of the temporal flow of events that accompanies it (12). She points out that
there is frequently a reordering of events in a traumatized child's
mind, such that events actually happening *after* an occurrence
are perceived to have happened *before* it, giving rise to a sense of
the ability to predict the future. These "powers," however, develop only after the traumatic event and because of it. This construct will be seen in Joseph's practice of crystal gazing—the
ability to stare at a fixed point or object until consciousness is altered and vivid hallucinations supervene (13). This practice has
been described by Nemiah as highly prevalent among those suffering from dissociative disorders. Traumatized children typically
possess an illusory sense of being gifted.

Aside from the general patterns of behavior seen in traumatized children, it is important to recognize that surgical operations themselves produce a set of specific emotional stresses in
young boys. Empirically, one thinks of surgery as one of society's
noblest fusions of art and science. But the hard reality, having little to do with art or science, is that *a surgical operation is, at its
core, a violent act performed by one person upon another.* In
a way, the art and science (anesthesia included) are merely disguises in their own right that protect patient and surgeon alike
from the reality of the interaction.

Adults and children are likely to perceive this violent act in
fundamentally different ways. An informed adult will usually accept the anxiety and discomfort of an operation as a tolerable
trade-off for an anticipated benefit. Only if things go awry will the

adult recognize the violence for what it is. In this circumstance, the adult often construes the event as some sort of *assault* ("Members of the jury, this butcher . . ."). But the small child has much less capacity to accept the trade-off. Instead, the child will more likely interpret any deliberate violence inflicted by an adult male not as assault, but as *punishment*. As Gerald Pearson writes of a child undergoing surgery:

> He does not know what has happened to him, and he postulates the worst possible. He has fantasies as to what did happen to him which are far in excess of the actual facts; . . . fantasies [that] make him entirely different from any one else in the world.
>
> He may become very angry and desire to hurt and destroy the person or persons (the physicians or his parents) who were responsible for his fright. This anger may . . . [displace] the fear by playing that he is performing the operation on another child. If the anger is not openly expressed, either motorially or verbally, its presence can be detected in the child's dream life.
>
> *Such fantasies and reactions . . . occur in all children who are subjected to an operation* and occur to some extent even if the operative procedure is explained to the child and he is allowed to verbalize and discuss all his ideas and fears. (14) [emphasis added]

Operations such as Joseph's are known to be especially troubling if immobilization is required after the procedure. Children studied during such immobilization have been typically found to develop a connection between their immobilization and a need to "atone" for some naughtiness (15). Joseph not only was immobilized but experienced a sense of banishment. The aggregate of circumstances could not have been worse.

Pain itself varies dramatically among children, determined in large measure by the degree to which the pain is charged with psychic significance. Since children, in particular, tend to adopt pain readily into their world of fantasy and ascribe to it some force existing in the fantasy, it is a fair assumption that Joseph Smith, Jr.'s pain was at the top end of the scale with the issues on which it probably centered. As Anna Freud has stated, "Pain augmented by anxiety . . ., even if slight in itself, represents a major event in the child's life and is remembered a long time afterward, the memory being frequently accompanied by phobic defenses against its possible return" (16).

Unfortunately, children have the additional difficulty of trying to sort out the underlying disease from the treatment that alleviates it. They must passively submit both to the disease inside and to the suffering imposed from without by caregivers. In "certain instances," these treatments, says Anna Freud, "with their high emotional significance, may even be the decisive ones in causing a child's psychological breakdown during illness, or in determining the aftereffects" (17).

The theme of castration appears as a regular part of male childhood fantasies surrounding all surgical operations after the age of three. This fear is at the core of all ideas of being attacked or overwhelmed. Thus Joseph's perception of his surgery as an aggressive, violent punishment would have been experienced on some level as retribution for his age-appropriate, guilt-ridden fantasy.

Joseph's fear of such dismemberment need not have been related to a direct assault on his genitalia. In fact, psychoanalyst Helene Deutsch points out that operations on peripheral organs are actually more likely to produce castration anxiety than are operations on more inner organs, including the genitalia (18). Anna Freud holds the same view:

> Whatever part of the body is operated on will take over by displacement the role of an injured genital part. The actual experience of the operation lends a feeling of reality to the repressed fantasies, thereby multiplying the anxieties connected with them. (19)

In this regard, it is important to note the centrality of the anger that Joseph seemed to direct against his father (and toward his father's accomplice surgeons) who had "punished" him so brutally in his operations. Such feelings themselves toward his father should hardly have been unfamiliar to Joseph at a young age, nor should they have been to any boy. But their repetitive reinforcement in such a savage and agonizing drama in the real world of his own bedroom by his abandoning mother and twelve dismembering fathers (including his real one) aborted to some degree the normal progression of his childhood development. Under normal circumstances, Joseph should have been able to resolve as well as any other boy those conflicted feelings toward his father, but not after the horror of the operations. Those murderous thoughts would thereafter simmer beneath the surface until something triggered their release. On reemergence, they would strike not at the real father, but instead at some figure of authority who in some way resembled that father—a governor, judge, preacher, lawyer, physician, journalist, or scholar.

Joseph would express his anger in several ways. He might recapitulate the circumstances of the operation by adopting the "victim" role in reenacting elements of the trauma, as he did in many of his speeches. In this vein, he seems to have developed a genius for getting himself attacked by all-male mobs in reenactments of the original trauma, perhaps creating new chances to master the earlier event. Alternatively, he might reverse the original scenario of the trauma and take the role of perpetrator, wielding the knife himself and brandishing it against his enemies in play, in literary fantasy, or in military uniform. And finally, rage and self-destruction might erupt impulsively when he encountered frustration. This sort of reaction will be seen in a final episode of rage that would cost him his life.

But the concept of "ambivalence" must not be ignored. With all of the fear, hatred, and loathing that the trauma had engendered in Joseph toward his father, he would bestow an equal aliquot of love, reverence, and admiration. The internalization of these exalted qualities of his father may have been the origin of his godlike view of himself.

One of these two views of his father (and perforce of himself) seemed to rule from within at any one moment to govern the limits of his behavior—but not both at once. This "splitting" of his father (or another male individual with power), again typical of traumatized children, would be manifest in fantasy as well as in reality. While one view of his father would be consciously recognized at all times, the other would be lurking beneath the surface, at risk for erupting under the proper stimulus. Joseph's behavior would often be hard to understand.

Further distinction needs to be made between children and adults in their respective reactions to trauma. Such a distinction is critical in studying Joseph Smith, Jr., because one such event occurred in his childhood and the other, an event related to the death of his brother, during late adolescence. Ordinarily, according to Robert Simon (20), dissociation does not occur as a reaction to trauma beyond the age of seven. A more typical pattern after this age is the frightening "flashback," as often experienced by combat veterans following their return to civilian life. However, an established pattern of dissociation, such as Joseph evidently developed in response to his operations, could in fact allow later stresses to flow into this more puerile pattern.

Two years after Joseph's operation and while he was still on crutches, Mount Tamboro exploded in a colossal eruption in the East Indies, vaporizing 40 cubic miles of rock. As this debris slowly distributed itself around the world, the sun's rays didn't penetrate as well to the rocky New England landscape as in previous years. Snow fell in June. There were killing frosts in July. Famine loomed. Thousands of New England farmers abandoned their rocky plots of land with their frozen crops in 1816 for the promise of better prospects in the black soil of New York and Ohio. The Smith family was among them. At the age of ten, Joseph, Jr. left his childhood farm home in Norwich, Vermont, for New York State with a few possessions and considerable emotional baggage.

That all the features of Joseph's emerging adult personality were well in place at this time is exemplified in his account of his memories of the journey. The following recounting appears immediately after his description of his operation in the *Manuscript History of the Church*. The centrality of the childhood trauma in the dynamics of his personality is subtly portrayed in the narrative:

After I began to get about on crutches till I started for the State of New York where my father had gone for the purpose of preparing a place for the removal of his family, which he affected by sending a man after us by the name of Caleb Howard, who, after he had started on, the journey with my mother and family spent the money he had received of my father by drinking and gambling, etc—We fell in with a family by the name of Gates who were travelling west, and Howard drove me from the waggon and made me travel in my weak state through the snow 40 miles per day for several days, during which time I suffered the most excrutiating weariness and pain, and all this that Mr. Howard might enjoy the society of two of Mr. Gates daughters which he took on the wagon where I should hive Rode, and thus he continued to do day after day through the Journey and when my brothers remonstrated with Mr. Howard for his treatment to me, he would knock them down with the butt of his whipp. —When we arrived at Utica, N. York[,] Howard threw the goods out of the waggon into the street and attempted to run away with the Horses and waggon, but my mother seized the horses by the reign, and[,] calling witnesses[,] forbid his taking them away as they were her propirty. On our way from Utica, I was left to ride on the last sleigh in the company, (the Gates family were in sleighs) but when that came up I was knocked down by the driver, one of Gate's Sons, and left to wollow in my blood until a stranger came along, picked me up, and carried me to the Town of Palmyra. —Howard having spent all our funds[,] My Mother was compelled to pay our landlords bills from Utica to Palmyra in bits of cloth, clothing, etc. the last payment being made with [drops?] taken from Sister Sophrona's [ears?], for that purpose. Although the snow was generally deep through the country during this Journey we performed the whole on wheels, except the first two days when we were accompanied by My Mother's mother, grandmother, Lydia Mack[,] who was injured by the upsetting of the Sleigh, and not wishing to accompany her friends west, tarried by the way with her friends in Vermont, and we soon heard of her death suffering that she never recovered from the injury received by the overturn of the Sleigh. (21)

In this account a kind of direct reenactment of Joseph's victimization in his operations can be identified. Early in the tale is seen an evil-father representation, Caleb Howard. Joseph's ambivalence toward his real father is implied at the beginning of the recounting, when Joseph relates that 1) this scoundrel, Howard, was imposed on the family through specific selection by his *evil-father* and 2) his *good-father's* hard-earned cash had been squandered in sinful deeds by Howard. This simultaneous "splitting" of his father into two opposite and powerful images will reappear over and over in Joseph's narratives. Next, he describes his persecution and injury as he is kicked out of his rightful throne in the wagon into the snow, where he must limp in pain 40 miles a day. Why is he thus victimized? So that his powerful rival may enjoy the pleasures of the Gates girls, who are sitting "where I should hive Rode." When protests are made, children are beaten with the "butt of his whipp." Perhaps Joseph, Jr. experienced a wish fulfillment when his mother sent the evil Howard away, interpreting her actions as a sign that she preferred the affection of her son. When Joseph starts afresh, another evil-father substitute, someone again connected with those Gates girls, bloodies him again. In the final lines Joseph complains that the evil-father substitute added an extra measure of suffering by causing the death of Joseph's grandmother.

In Joseph's "abandonment," only some passing stranger (read "good-father") can save him. As Leonard Shengold has noted,

> If the child must turn to the very parent who inflicts abuse and who is felt as bad . . ., [the child] must register the parent, *delusionally,* as good. Only the mental image of a good parent who will rescue can help the child deal with the terrifying intensity of fear and rage that is the effect of the tormenting experiences. (22)

The facts of the episode as related by Joseph can be partially corroborated in his mother's description of the same event (although, as before, she places herself in a more "in charge" posture). But there is an unmistakable flavor of persecution by a powerful male overlying a recurring oedipal theme that characterizes the spin of Joseph's narrative. Such persecution occurs twice in a single short vignette. There must have been hundreds of other memorable events of all flavors that took place in Joseph's middle childhood, and even on the journey to upstate New York. In his autobiography, however, immediately after describing his childhood operation, Joseph chooses to share only this grim and sordid tale of repetitive persecution and betrayal by powerful and brutish males. By selecting this event, Joseph reveals much about the nature of the brooding in his mind and what sort of key or password of daily experience will open his mind's locked file of dissociated memory.

The grim themes of the story are identical to those that will be seen repetitively in the main bulk of his writings over his lifetime: helplessness, victimization, death, betrayal, randomness, trauma, hand weapons, shame, blood against a white surface, and evil-father representations. Also evident is the recurring theme of his painful journey as a victim, identical to what Joseph had experienced in his overland "banishment" to the seashore. Any modern fifth-grade teacher who received such a paper as this from a pupil would be negligent if he or she did not alert the guidance counselor to help a troubled boy. These themes of persecution will be met again and again as Joseph narrates his interpersonal relationships with the many, many Caleb Howards yet to be encountered.

Notes

1. Smith J: *Manuscript History of the Church*, Book A-1. Salt Lake City, LDS Church Historian's Office, 1838, p. 131. See also Durham RC: "Joseph Smith's Own Story of a Serious Childhood Illness." *BYU Studies* 10(Summer):480–482, 1970.
2. Terr L: *Unchained Memories: True Stories of Traumatic Memories, Lost and Found.* New York, Basic Books, 1994, p. 87.
3. Terr L: *Too Scared to Cry: Psychic Trauma in Childhood.* New York, Harper & Row, 1990, p. 113.

4. Smith LM: *Biographical Sketches of Joseph Smith the Prophet and His Progenitors for Many Generations.* Liverpool, S. W. Richards, 1853 [reprinted New York, Arno Press, 1969], p. 85.

5. Shengold L: *Soul Murder: The Effects of Childhood Abuse and Deprivation.* New Haven, CT, Yale University Press, 1989, p. 229.

6. Waites EA: *Trauma and Survival: Post-Traumatic Dissociative Disorders in Women.* New York, W. W. Norton, 1993, p. 204.

7. Terr L: *Too Scared to Cry,* p. 255.

8. Nemiah JC: "Dissociative Disorders (Hysterical Neuroses, Dissociative Type)," in *Comprehensive Textbook of Psychiatry/V,* 5th Edition, Vol. 2. Edited by Kaplan HI, Sadock BJ. Baltimore, Williams & Wilkins, 1989, pp. 1028–1044; see p. 1034.

9. Lightner MER: "Remarks." Given at Brigham Young University, April 14, 1905. Typescript BYU, LDS Historical Department, Salt Lake City. See also Newell LK, Avery VT: *Mormon Enigma: Emma Hale Smith.* Garden City, NY, Doubleday & Co., 1984, p. 31.

10. Stevenson E: *Autobiography of Edward Stevenson.* Salt Lake City, LDS Church Archives, 1891, p. 20. Quoted in Vogel D (ed): *Early Mormon Documents,* Vol. 1. Salt Lake City, Signature Books, 1996, p. 38.

11. Terr L: *Unchained Memories,* p. 86.

12. Terr L: *Too Scared to Cry,* pp. 146–167.

13. Nemiah J: "Dissociative Disorders (Hysterical Neuroses, Dissociative Type)," p. 1034.

14. Pearson GHJ: "Effect of Operative Procedures on the Emotional Life of the Child." *American Journal of Diseases of Children* 62:716–729, 1941; see pp. 720–721.

15. Bergmann T: "Observations of Children's Reactions to Motor Restraint." *The Nervous Child* 4:318–328, 1945.

16. Freud A: "The Role of Bodily Illness in the Mental Life of Children." *Psychoanalytic Study of the Child* 7:69–81, 1952; see p. 76.

17. Ibid., p. 70.

18. Deutsch H: "Some Psychoanalytic Observations in Surgery." *Psychosomatic Medicine* 4:105–115, 1942.

19. Freud A: "The Role of Bodily Illness in the Mental Life of Children," pp. 74–75.

20. Simon RI: *Bad Men Do What Good Men Dream: A Forensic Psychiatrist Illuminates the Darker Side of Human Behavior.* Washington, DC, American Psychiatric Press, 1996, p. 187.

21. Smith J: *Manuscript History of the Church,* Book A-1, pp. 131–132.

22. Shengold L: *Soul Murder,* p. 26.

Chapter Four

The Pleasure of Treasure

There is a common myth that appears in nearly all cultures: that of the discovery of secret treasure. As outlined by psychoanalyst Selma Fraiberg,

> Typically the treasure story follows this pattern: A poor boy or man accidentally discovers a secret which leads him to buried treasure or to the acquisition of great wealth. Usually the treasure is the stolen loot of a bandit, a pirate or an evil sorcerer; it may be buried in the ground or in a mysterious cavern. The hero obtains secret knowledge of the treasure either through a conniving and evil person who wishes to use the innocent hero for a tool, or through the accidental "overhearing" or "overseeing" of an event which betrays the secret, or through the acquisition of a magic formula or device or a map or code. Usually, too, the hero must overcome an evil opponent who seeks the treasure. The treasure is success-

fully won by the hero who vanquishes his enemies, marries a beautiful princess, or brings wealth and prestige to his mother, elevating her from her humble and impoverished station. (1)

Fraiberg also notes:

"Mother is unhappy," such fantasies begin, often enough with some truth. "Father is poor and there is never enough money." Or: "Father does not make her happy. . . . If I were rich I would give all my money to mother. I would give her everything she wanted. And she would love *me* best! But I am not rich. . . . Supposing. . . ." And now the daydream proper begins. "How can I get rich? . . . I am digging in the garden one day when I see a little tin box. . . . I am walking down the street one day when I see a purse. . . . I find a scrap of paper and I am just about to throw it away when I see something written on it . . . ." There are endless variations to such daydreams. (2)

Regardless of whether the scene is a desert island or a mysterious castle, the following elements are always present: 1) a "fearless and honest fellow" who 2) accidentally discovers the secret, 3) outwits those who would also try to steal it, and 4) opens and claims the treasure. A common psychological theme of childhood runs through all such myths across many ages and cultures—one which has been repressed and is no longer available to the consciousness of the author or the audience. Only the excitement in the telling and listening betrays the communication and the connection.

Fraiberg makes the psychoanalytic argument that the myth of treasure-seeking is, at its core, an expression of the repressed memories of the universal childhood oedipal fantasy. The goal of triumphing over father and possessing mother is achieved through the sexual symbols in this universal fantasy. In Fraiberg's words:

These tales of the buried treasure and discovery of great wealth are among the oldest daydreams of the race. These are the longings of childhood which live on in the uncon-

scious memory of the grown man. Their ageless appeal derives from the universal and perennial mystery which
confounds the child in his first investigations of origins. In
every life there is this momentous discovery of the secret
through an accidental touching or an observation, a revelation of the "magic" of the genitals. And always there has been
a magician with greater powers and a secret knowledge
which is denied to a poor boy. There is the childhood mystery of "the place" where the treasure is hidden, the mysterious cavern which has no door, the hidden place deep under
ground. And there is the unwavering belief of the child that
if he should have the magician's magic lamp, the pirate's
map, the key to the treasure, the knowledge of "the place,"
he could win for himself this treasure of treasures. In this
ageless daydream of childhood, the poor boy who has nothing steals the magician's secret, the pirate's map, and outwits the powerful opponent who stands between him and
the treasure. (3)

Treasure-seeking was especially popular among the rural
poor in early nineteenth-century New England. The common tal-
ismans for discovering it—the divining rod (like that of Joseph
Smith, Sr.), the seer-stones, and the magic daggers used for drawing circles on the ground—all shared the symbolism of the magical devices Fraiberg has described. But as Fawn Brodie describes
in her biography of Joseph Smith, Jr.,

> . . . where the Green Mountains yielded nothing but an oc-
> casional cache of counterfeit money, western New York and
> Ohio were rich in Indian relics. Hundreds of burial mounds
> dotted the landscape, filled with skeletons and artifacts of
> stone, copper, and sometimes beaten silver. There were
> eight such tumuli within twelve miles of the Smith farm. (4)

Joseph Smith, Jr. and his father became deeply involved in
treasure-seeking sometime during their first three years in
Palmyra, New York. As a number of individuals in the area were
using seer-stones, Joseph took great interest in these devices. The
most notable of the "glass-lookers" in the region was the young

woman Sally Chase, whom Joseph begged his parents to let him
visit at the age of 13 to see her glassy green stone:

> He did so, and was permitted to look in the glass, which was
> placed in a hat to exclude the light. He was greatly surprised
> to see but one thing, which was a small stone, a great way off.
> It soon became luminous, and dazzled his eyes, and after
> a short time it became as intense as the mid-day sun. He said
> that the stone was under the roots of a tree or shrub as large
> as his arm . . . He borrowed an old ax and a hoe, and re-
> paired to the tree. With some labor and exertion he found
> the stone. (5)

As noted in the previous chapter, this sort of crystal gazing is
seen frequently among individuals who carry dissociated memories of past trauma. Staring at a fixed point such as an imperfection
in glass can often induce a hypnotic state in traumatized individuals, with visual hallucinations of just the sort related in this passage,
opening the door to the "split off" world of trauma-related memories. This face-in-the-hat method appeared to be Joseph's favorite
method of using his stone. Although the sexual symbolism of this
act should not be overlooked, he may also have favored this
method because the element of darkness facilitated his entry into
a trance. (Does this further suggest that young Joseph might have
been blindfolded in some way during his operation?)

This description of crystal gazing is an important confirmation
of the function of the dissociation mechanism in Joseph's mind,
wherein the self-induction of the trance is illustrated. In this case
the significance of the specific content may only be guessed at,
though Fraiberg's analysis of the treasure hunt as a fantasy of
childhood sexuality offers a clue. As in Fraiberg's description of
the universal myth, Joseph's treasure was found in a hole beneath
a tree. Fraiberg notes the sexual symbolism of these elements, an
observation that is relevant to the nature of the universal age-
specific fantasy against which Joseph's childhood trauma seems
to have occurred.

Ultimately armed with three seer-stones, Joseph, Jr. indulged
his treasure-seeking fantasies to their fullest. Usually accompanied by others of like interest, including his father, he gained local

fame as a "peeper," directing and guiding diggers in their search for riches of gold, silver, and treasures. Staring into the stones until the trance came on, he described his hallucinations to his followers. It is fair to assume that these followers were as struck by the "search light" of his white countenance and his "transparency" as was Mary Elizabeth Rollins Lightner, who had described Joseph, Jr. in such terms during his later oratory (see opening to Chapter 1).

The loose fraternity of rodsmen involved in the treasure-digging activities appears to have had some common roots as far back as when Joseph, Jr. was in Vermont and even earlier through family ties in Connecticut. Included in this murky group was Luman Walter, a physician-cum-clairvoyant and "vagabond fortune-teller," who once read aloud to his followers in an exotic tongue from an ancient Indian record about the location of hidden treasure (but which was actually a Latin copy of Cicero's *Orations*). Also involved were Nathaniel and Justus Winchell, who had been "warned out" of Middletown, Vermont, during the bizarre Wood Scrape affair mentioned in Chapter 2. These men and others, as well as his own father, served as mentors for Joseph Smith, Jr. in his growing immersion in treasure-seeking (4, 5). But while historical accounts of the integrity of these companions are almost always couched in derogatory terms (with some apparent justification), Joseph's own psychodynamics may have been quite different. Nonetheless, the future prophet grew to become the most renowned "glass-looker" in the Palmyra area.

The rituals of treasure-digging that Joseph led in the rural moonlight of New York State brimmed with his own familiar themes of violence, spilled blood, death, threatening evil fathers, sexual symbolism, and assault by the sword. In one set of Joseph, Jr.'s instructions, the diggers were "to stick a parcel of large stakes in the ground, several rods around, in a circular form" over the spot where the treasure was supposedly buried. "A messenger was then sent to Palmyra to procure a polished sword: after which, Samuel F. Lawrence, with a drawn sword in his hand, marched around to guard any assault which his Satanic majesty might be disposed to make" (6). In another ritual, "[a] black sheep should be taken on to the ground where the treasures were concealed—that after cutting its throat, it should be led around a circle while bleeding. This being done, the wrath of the evil spirit would be appeased . . ." (7).

In these blood rituals of violence may be seen disguised reenactments of Joseph's brutal trauma. As with the tale of Caleb Howard, the themes are grim and repetitive. The only difference is the fact that Joseph has now reversed the roles, as is typical in the dream life of boys after surgery. Now he himself wields the scalpel and holds the power. Victimization has become triumph. Although he may have inherited some of the plot lines from his mentors, he selected the elements for each dramatization, he produced them, he directed them, and he was certainly the most gratified member of their audience. As with Stephen King, the horrible event in Joseph's childhood seems to have driven his creative expression through fantasies by which was reenacted literally that which he could not consciously remember.

Indeed, Terr has commented that such posttraumatic "play" often takes the form of forbidden games conducted under a cloak of secrecy with a contagious level of fascination that draws many eager participants. It is as though Joseph wanted to make others feel the emotions of horror he himself had experienced. These ritual dramatizations of his unceasing conflict reappeared in repetitive fashion from farmstead to farmstead in upstate New York. Although at this stage in his life he was successful in enticing only a few superstitious farmers to assist him in acting out the conflicts arising from his childhood trauma, the treasure-seeking rituals would serve as the preliminary rehearsals for much bigger stages and ever more complex ceremonies and structures to come. The drawn sword, the symbol of the nightmare of his past, would yet slash permanent scars into the face of the American frontier, even as it ultimately impaled its bearer.

But as Joseph would discover repeatedly throughout his life, the overt expressions of this segregated appendage of his mind would often not be taken kindly by the local citizenry. His first known confrontation with this painful fact occurred in connection with these very money-digging activities. As his reputation for clairvoyance had spread far beyond the environs of Palmyra, he was invited at the age of 16 or 17 to assist in locating a treasure near Harmony, Pennsylvania, in the Susquehanna Valley. The digging never achieved success despite two or three years of sporadic efforts, into 1825. Joseph, Jr.'s father accompanied him during much of the digging. The principal enthusiast and paymaster of these ventures was Josiah Stowel, of South Bainbridge, New York, an elderly farmer who believed deeply in Joseph's magical powers. In 1825 the digging centered on or near the property of Isaac Hale, another transplanted Vermont farmer. Hale described Joseph's activities and demeanor as follows:

> . . . his occupation was that of seeing, or pretending to see by means of a stone placed in his hat, and his hat closed over his face. In this way he pretended to discover minerals and hidden treasure. His appearance at this time, was that of a careless young man—not very well educated and *very saucy and insolent to his father.* . . . Young Smith gave the "money-diggers" great encouragement, at first, but when they had arrived in digging to near the place where he had stated an immense treasure would be found—he said the enchantment was so powerful that he could not see. They then became discouraged, and soon after dispersed. (8) (emphasis added)

Again, although the skeptical tone of Hale's remarks suggests deceit on Joseph's part, it was perhaps just as likely that Joseph's dissociative trance had become so terrifying for some reason that he had become genuinely incapacitated. This speculation will be readdressed in Chapter 6.

Joseph tarried in the region of Stowel's farm into 1826, in part because of his interest in Hale's daughter Emma. But in March, one of Stowel's nephews, Peter Bridgman, acting on behalf of Stowel's sons, who were watching part of their inheritance disappear into Joseph's pockets, swore out a warrant for Joseph's arrest as an impostor and disorderly person. The Vagrant Act of New York State had brought numerous types of vagrancy under the legal heading "disorderly persons," including "all persons pretending to have skill in physiognomy, palmistry, or the like crafty sciences, or pretending to tell fortunes, or to discover where lost goods may be found" (9). The court record of *People of State of*

New York vs. Joseph Smith (March 20, 1826) unintentionally reveals considerable insight into the scope and pattern of Joseph's
dissociative trances, indicating that

> Prisoner . . . [s]ays that he . . . had a certain stone, which he
> had occasionally looked at to determine where hidden
> treasures in the bowels of the earth were; that he professed
> to tell in this manner where gold-mines were a distance un-
> der ground, and had looked for Mr. Stowel several times,
> and informed him where he could find those treasures, and
> Mr. Stowel had been engaged in digging for them; that at
> Palmyra he pretended to tell, by looking at this stone, where
> coined money was buried in Pennsylvania, and while at
> Palmyra he had frequently ascertained in that way where lost
> property was, of various kinds; that he has occasionally been
> in the habit of looking through this stone to find lost prop-
> erty for three years, but of late had pretty much given it
> up on account of its injuring his health, especially his
> eyes—made them sore; that he did not solicit business of
> this kind, and had always rather declined having anything to
> do with this business. (10)

Stowel's own testimony bespoke a firm personal belief in the
powers of the young man:

> Josiah Stowel sworn. . . . [He said] that prisoner had told by
> means of this stone where a Mr. Bacon had buried money;
> that he and prisoner had been in search of it; that prisoner
> said that it was in a certain root of a stump five feet from sur-
> face of the earth and with it would be found a tail-feather;
> that said Stowel and prisoner thereupon commenced dig-
> ging, found a tail-feather, but money was gone; that he sup-
> posed that money moved down . . . (11)

Others at the trial testified skeptically of Joseph's professed
ability to read books with his stone:

> Arad Stowel sworn. Says that he went to see whether pris-
> oner could convince him that he possessed the skill that he
> professed to have, upon which prisoner laid a book upon
> a white cloth, and proposed looking through another stone

which was white and transparent; hold the stone to the candle, turn his back to book and read. The deception appeared so palpable, that he went off disgusted. (12)

Another witness testified of Joseph's claims of visions of Indians and violence, a theme already well developed in Joseph's vivid sublimations:

Jonathan Thompson says that prisoner was requested to look for Yeomans for chest of money. . . . Smith looked in hat while there, and when very dark, and told how the chest was situated. After digging several feet, struck upon something sounding like a board or plank. Prisoner would not look again, pretending that he was alarmed the last time that he looked, on account of the circumstances relating to the trunk being buried came all fresh to his mind; that the last time that he looked, he discovered distinctly the two Indians who buried the trunk; that a quarrel ensued between them, and that one of said Indians was killed by the other, and thrown in the hole beside of the trunk, to guard it, as he supposed. Thompson says that he believes in the prisoner's professed skill; that the board which he struck his spade upon was probably the chest, but, on account of an enchantment, the trunk kept settling away from under them while digging . . .
And thereupon the Court finds the defendant guilty. (13)

Because he was a minor, Joseph was apparently not sentenced but instead was permitted to take "leg bail" and get out of town. A justice of the peace who would preside at a later local trial of Joseph wrote that "Jo, was not seen in our town for 2 Years or more (except in Dark Corners)" (14).

The flavor of Joseph's own testimony ("had pretty much given it up," "did not solicit business of this kind," "had always rather declined having anything to do with this business") suggests that he accepted his humiliation with some shame over his conduct and with the expectation of punishment. Lawyers and justices would in the process become for him a permanently loathed class of powerful fatherlike enemies against whom he would rail bitterly in his speeches and writings for the remainder of his life.

There would be more such groups. But such an unpleasant diversion in the real world could hardly extinguish the fire for treasure-seeking glowing in the special place in Joseph's mind. The humiliation would merely shift the modus operandi.

In the meantime Joseph found himself confronting another father-substitute whose rivalry would taste of a more familiar flavor. His amorous attentions were not at all welcomed by Emma Hale's burly father, Isaac, who, soon after his initial cautious participation in Joseph's money-digging, had turned contemptuous. A request for Emma's hand in marriage brought a flat refusal because the young suitor "followed a business that I could not approve" (15). But Isaac was often absent on hunting forays, and Joseph took advantage of one such opportunity to elope with Emma, "rescuing" her from her tyrannical keeper. They returned to the Smith home near Palmyra and moved in. Finding it necessary to make a brief journey back to the Hale home several months later to gather some of Emma's possessions, they hired a wagon whose driver later related the scene of the confrontation between Joseph and Isaac:

> His father-in-law (Mr. Hale) addressed Joseph, in a flood of tears: "You have stolen my daughter and married her. I had much rather have followed her to her grave. You spend your time in digging for money—pretend to see in a stone, and thus try to deceive people." Joseph wept, and acknowledged he could not see in a stone now, nor never could; and that his former pretensions in that respect, were all false. He then promised to give up his old habits of digging for money and looking into stones. (16)

In this instance, as in the trial a few months before, Joseph again reacted passively to condemnation at the hands of a father-substitute. He overtly denied the behavior that had been driven from within as he surrendered to humiliation. Could it be that in the return to Hale, Joseph somehow "contrived" this scene of assault as another reenactment in order to give himself another chance to master his early trauma?

A third episode of reactive disapproval from the community must have shaken Joseph as well. He was 17 years of age when his

oldest brother Alvin died suddenly in some form of intraab-
dominal catastrophe in his twenty-fifth year. According to Lucy's
description, an autopsy demonstrated that he had died of upper-
gastrointestinal obstruction from an overdose of calomel (a mer-
curous cathartic) prescribed by a physician other than the trusted
family doctor. After several days of vomiting, probably exacer-
bated by the purgatives administered at follow-up visits by doctors, he would likely have died of the consequences of low
blood-potassium levels, possible infection, or whatever other in-
traabdominal misfortune (most likely appendicitis or pancreati-
tis) had in fact occurred. The bitterness was deepened when
Reverend Stockton, the minister who preached the funeral sermon for the unchurched Alvin, "intimated very strongly that he
had gone to hell" (17).

And finally, months later, a rumor evidently began to circulate
that Alvin's body had been exhumed and dissected, presumably
for some necromantic reason related to the occult treasure-
digging practices of young Joseph and his family members.
Joseph, Sr. therefore unearthed the coffin, inspected the undis-
turbed body, and placed the following ad in the local *Wayne [New
York] Sentinel*:

TO THE PUBLIC: Whereas reports have been industriously
put in circulation that my son, Alvin, has been removed
from the place of his interment and dissected; which reports every person possessed of human sensibility must
know are peculiarly calculated to harrow up the mind of
a parent and deeply wound the feelings of relations, I, with
some of my neighbors this morning repaired to the grave,
and removing the earth, found the body, which had not
been disturbed. This method is taken for the purpose of sat-
isfying the minds of those who have put it in circulation,
that it is earnestly requested that they would desist therefrom; and that it is believed by some that they have been
stimulated more by desire to injure the reputation of certain persons than by a philanthropy for the peace and welfare of myself and friends.

(Signed) Joseph Smith
Palmyra, September 25, 1824 (18)

Such a cascade of highly charged events surrounding Alvin's death must have had enormous impact on the fragile psyche of Joseph Smith, Jr. His presumed background mélange of feelings—awe, affection, and rivalry—toward his oldest brother must have resulted in a confused mix of sadness and guilt at the unexpected death. Was Alvin a kind of auxiliary parent for Joseph as older siblings often are? Did the combined "betrayals" of two more father-substitutes in the persons of a substitute physician and the condescending Reverend Stockton help to frame Joseph's final image of Alvin into a saintly visage? At any rate, the evils of "doctor-craft" and "priest-craft" would be forever added to Joseph's growing list of contemptible father-substitute groups. Certainly the sense of humiliation and victimization he must have felt over the rumor of grave robbing should have increased the intensity of his conflict. He would be greatly troubled by Alvin's death, and the event would flow into his complex inner turmoil as further fuel for the potent driving forces of his behavior. This critically important event will be reexamined in Chapter 6 as subsequent clues in the biographical record make it more comprehensible as a factor in Joseph's behavior.

In the meantime, Joseph's sublimated world of fantasy was becoming ever more structured. Originally a disjointed mass of grim and violent daydream images following his trauma, Joseph's fantasies were becoming integrated into a more coordinated framework. His environment provided some exciting possibilities for scenes and backdrops, and the stories of others were worked into an increasingly interconnected plotline. In particular, the numerous Indian mounds in his neighborhood and the widespread speculation in the local newspapers about the nature and origin of the Moundbuilders made their way into the structure of his fantasies. Lucy recalls her son in his teens relating these fantasies to the family:

> During our evening conversations, Joseph would occasionally give us some of the most amusing recitals that could be imagined. He would describe the ancient inhabitants of this continent, their dress, mode of travelling, and the animals upon which they rode; their cities, their buildings, with every

particular; their mode of warfare; and also their religious
worship. This he would do with as much ease, seemingly, as
if he had spent his whole life with them. (19)

(Not his whole life, Lucy—just since the age of seven.)

The contributions from the local lore were numerous. In
1818 the *Palmyra Register* had speculated that the Moundbuilders had been "doubtless killed in battle and hastily buried" (20).
The *Western Farmer,* another Palmyra newspaper, had reported
in 1821 (when Joseph was 15) that "several brass plates," along
with skeletons and pottery shards, had been unearthed by diggers
on the Erie Canal (21). The *Palmyra Herald* had stated in 1823
that "what wonderful catastrophe destroyed the first inhabitants
is beyond the researches of the best scholar and greatest antiquar-
ian" (22). Joseph related to a friend that he had heard of a history
of the Indians being found in Canada at the base of a hollow tree
(always under the tree, says Fraiberg).

The local mysteries melded with the family passion for
treasure-digging and Joseph's already-formed fantasy world in
a grand fusion—the "discovery" of a history of the Moundbuilders. It would be unearthed through Joseph's gift of clairvoyance
and be translated by his ability to read books with his stone, and
would embody the complex sublimated world of fantasies still
bubbling up in his dissociations into an increasingly structured
daydream cosmos.

Although many interpretations of the historical narrative are
possible, Fraiberg's schema is especially helpful. There appears to
be a striking congruency between its sexualized theme and Joseph's
own treasure-seeking tale in all of the disparate versions of the
story in the biographical record. As Parley Chase, one of Joseph's
neighbors, stated, "In regard to their Gold Bible speculation, they
scarcely ever told two stories alike" (23). But since all of the accounts have the same elements, it will be of value to describe several. It should be remembered that all such myths contain the
elements of a poor, honest boy who accidentally discovers a secret, outwits those who would steal it, and opens and claims the
treasure so that he can satisfy his mother's needs.

The first such version of the story related that Joseph, Jr. had

divined the hiding place of some ancient gold plates that contained a short history of the previous inhabitants of America and
the locations of their buried treasure. He claimed that the plates
were in the charge of a spirit who would not give them up until
the proper moment. Joseph, Sr. was the source of many of his
son's statements about finding the plates at the time. Obadiah
Dogberry, the editor of the *Palmyra Reflector,* recalled in 1831
some of Joseph, Sr.'s comments, along with some of his own recollections:

> In the commencement, the imposture of the "Book of Mor-
> mon" had no regular plan or features. At a time when the
> money digging ardor was somewhat abated,[1] the elder
> Smith declared that his son Joe had seen the *spirit,* (which
> he then described as a little old man with a long beard,) and
> was informed that he (Jo) under certain circumstances,
> eventually should obtain great treasures, and that in due
> time he (the spirit) would furnish him (Jo) with a book,
> which would give an account of the ancient inhabitants (an-
> tideluvians) of this country, and where they had deposited
> their substance, consisting of costly furniture, etc., at the
> approach of the great deluge, which had ever since that time
> remained secure in his (the spirit's) charge, in large and
> spacious *chambers,* in sundry places in this vicinity, and
> these tidings corresponded precisely with revelations made
> to, and predictions made by the elder Smith a number of
> years before.
>   The time at length arrived, when young Joe was to re-
> ceive the book from the hand of the spirit, and he repaired
> accordingly, alone, and in the night time, to the woods in
> the rear of his father's house . . . and met the spirit as had
> been appointed. This rogue of a spirit who had baffled all
> the united efforts of the money diggers, (although they had
> tried many devices to gain his favor, and at one time sacri-
> ficed a barn yard fowl,) intended it would seem to play our
> prophet a similar trick on this occasion, for no sooner had
> he delivered the book according to promise, than he made

---

[1] This phrase would suggest that the time frame for this story would have
been after the Bainbridge trial in 1826.

a most desperate attempt to regain its possession. Our prophet, however, like a lad of true metal, stuck to his prize. . . . Joe retained his treasure and returned to the house with his father, much fatigued and injured. This tale in substance, was told at the time the event was said to have happened by both father and son, and is well recollected by many of our citizens. It will be borne in mind that no *divine* interposition had been *dreamed* of at the period. (24)

Again, one sees the fearless and honest fellow whose accidental discovery of a great treasure hidden in "large and spacious *chambers*" leads to the outwitting of the crafty "little old man with a long beard" (perhaps father-with-large-phallus?) in a triumphant battle for the great prize.

As to the ultimate purpose of the acquisition of this treasure, Joseph Capron recollected that

[a]t length, Joseph pretended to find the Gold plates. This scheme, he believed, would relieve the family from all pecuniary embarrassment. His father told me, that when the book was published, they would be enabled, from the profits of the work, to carry into successful operation the money-digging business. He gave me no intimation, at that time that the book was to be of a religious character, or that it had anything to do with revelation. He declared it to be a speculation, and said he "when it is completed, my family will be placed *on a level* above the generality of mankind"!! (25)

And thus would young Joseph fulfill Fraiberg's final tenet of the universal treasure-seeking fantasy.

There is another genre of stories in the historical record describing the acquisition of this treasure. These stories are more convoluted but no less in conformity with Fraiberg's schema. In this scenario, related nine years later by Joseph, Jr. himself, he was given the secret of the plates and their location in a thrice-repeated dream by an angel on Sunday night, September 21, 1823. The next morning an additional "vision" directed him to tell his father of his dream, an instruction that enabled Joseph to procure in his quest the essential imprimatur of his father. With the aid of his brown seer-stone he went to the nearby Hill Cumorah, where he and his father had performed numerous excavations previously, and found the plates in a stone box, along with a breastplate of armor and a pair of magic glasses consisting of two seer-stones in silver bows.

Keeping in mind Fraiberg's discussion of treasure discovery as a sexual fantasy and the female symbolism of the cavities in which treasure is hidden, the reader may assess any anatomic resemblance through Joseph Smith, Jr.'s own words as he described the "stone box" wherein he found the plates: "This stone was thick and rounding in the middle on the upper side, and thinner towards the edges, so that the middle part of it was visible above the ground, but the edge all around was covered with earth" (26).

The representation of the female genitalia as a receptacle or box in dream or fantasy is one of the most universal, according to Freud. The vulgar use of the term "box" to describe the vagina is present in many languages, including German, as Freud's own references to it attest (27).

(This seems not to have been Joseph's only instance of sexualization of his treasure box. Under oath in a civil trial, Leman Copley testified that Joseph had described to him that after completing his translation and returning the plates to an angel, he had an encounter in the woods:

> He [Joseph] discovered an old man dressed in ordinary gray apparel, sitting upon a log, having in his hand or near by, a small box. On approaching him, he asked him what he had in his box. To which the old man replied, that he had a MONKEY, and for five coppers he might see it. Joseph answered, that he would not give a cent to see a monkey, for he had seen a hundred of them. . . . Joseph then passed on . . . and finally asked the Lord the meaning of it. The Lord told him that the man he saw was MORONI, with the plates, and if he had given him the five coppers, he might have got his plates again. (28)

The passage is incomprehensible unless one is aware that the term "monkey" was a common nineteenth-century vulgarism for the female genitalia [29], as it is most unlikely that Joseph would have seen a single true simian, much less "a hundred," in the upstate New York of 1828.)

Joseph continues his narrative of uncovering his treasure in a suggestive description of plunder and discovery:

> Having removed the earth, I obtained a lever, which I got fixed under the edge of the stone, and with a little exertion raised it up. I looked in, and there indeed did I behold the plates, the Urim and Thummim, and the breastplate, as stated by the messenger. (30)

Joseph goes on with his story, from which can be inferred frustration (or tantalization, if one prefers):

> I made an attempt to take them out, but was forbidden by the messenger, and was again informed that the time for bringing them forth had not yet arrived, neither would it, until four years from that time; but he told me that I should come to that place precisely in one year from that time, and that he would there meet with me, and that I should continue to do so until the time should come for obtaining the plates. Accordingly, as I had been commanded, I went at the end of each year, and at each time I found the same messenger there, and received instruction and intelligence from him at each of our interviews . . . (31)

Certainly this powerful "messenger" would seem a formidable rival who would protect that prize from all but the cleverest aspirant. But according to Joseph, Sr., his son's first visit to the hill was yet more eventful. As related by Willard Chase:

> In the month of June, 1827, Joseph Smith, Sen., related to me the following story: That some years ago, a spirit had appeared to Joseph his son, in a vision, and informed him that in a certain place there was a record on plates of gold, and that he was the person that must obtain them, and this he must do in the following manner: On the 22nd of September, he must repair to the place where was deposited

this manuscript, dressed in black clothes, and riding a black horse with a switch tail, and demand the book in a certain name, and after obtaining it, he must go directly away, and neither lay it down nor look behind him. They accordingly fitted out Joseph with a suit of black clothes and borrowed a black horse. He repaired to the place of deposit and demanded the book which was in a stone box, unsealed, and so near the top of the ground that he could see one end of it, and raising it up, took out the book of gold; but fearing some one might discover where he got it, he laid it down to place back the top stone, as he found it; and turning round, to his surprise there was no book in sight. He again opened the box, and in it saw the book, and attempted to take it out but was hindered. He saw in the box something like a toad, which soon assumed the appearance of a man, and struck him on the side of the head.—Not being discouraged at trifles, he again stooped down and strove to take the book, when the spirit struck him again, and knocked him three or four rods. . . . After recovering from his fright, he enquired why he could not obtain the plates; to which the spirit made reply, because you have not obeyed your orders. He then enquired when he *could* have them, and was answered thus: come one year from this day, and bring with you your oldest brother, and you shall have them. . . . Before the expiration of the year, his oldest brother died: which the old man said was an *accidental providence*! (32)

Is Fraiberg's sexual theme cryptically displayed in Chase's version of the narrative? Joseph dresses in black and rides a black horse, presumably in order to favor concealment in his forbidden act. He finds and acquires the treasure of treasures in an unsealed cavity. However, panicky over the fear of discovery, he unhands his treasure momentarily, only to find that it has replaced itself in its rightful repository. But on this second occasion his manual efforts at again handling the delightsome treasure are thwarted by discovery. The toad who shares that repository and quickly metamorphoses into a rivalrous fatherlike visage takes umbrage at the intrusive trespass and has soon "knocked him three or four rods," keeping his own treasure where it rightfully belongs.

The "something like a toad" in this narrative has received

more than a little attention by Mormon historians. Quinn and others have speculated that reference was being made to a salamander, the creature often seen in fiery visage in occult tales, guarding treasure and communicating with humans. *Moron* was the scientific name for a poisonous salamander, and *Imoron* is an American Indian word for a poisonous creature (33). (The angel who had visited Joseph in his three dreams was named "Moroni.") On the other hand, the "fiery" association is in keeping with Fraiberg's recurring theme of the sexual symbolism of treasure-digging, which parallels the fire-producing lamp in the Aladdin tale and the similar fiery talisman in the treasure story "The Tinder Box" of Hans Christian Andersen.

Bettelheim points out (34), however, that frogs and salamanders have different connotations in fairy tales as manifestations of unconscious themes from childhood. The frog is for children a repugnant creature, representing in fairy tales the disgust children appropriately feel toward sexual matters; the subliminal message of the stories is that it is okay to feel disgust about sex until one is ready for it. This is in part the message of metamorphosis from puerile to mature existence, so well symbolized by the frog's transformation from tadpole to adult. A possible unconscious association between the frog and sex is further seen in the child's connection between the tacky, clammy sensations evoked by frogs and salamanders and the similar feelings attached to the sex organs. The message, as conveyed in tales in which kissing a frog provokes a glorious metamorphosis, is that sex may become beautiful if one can learn to approach it with maturity. That fearful issues haunted Joseph Smith's own sexuality is a theme that will be explored in Chapter 7.

Finally, an even more intriguing version of Joseph's sublimated fantasy is an account of the second visit to the hill on the following September, in 1824, as related much later by Joseph's mother Lucy. One might also listen for the same sexual theme hiding in this version of this visit, with its overtones of forbidden pleasure and punishment:

> Therefore, having arrived at the place, and uncovering the
> plates, he put forth his hand and took them up, but, as he

was taking them hence, the unhappy thought darted through his mind that probably there was something else in the box besides the plates, which would be of some pecuniary advantage to him. So, in the moment of excitement, he laid them down very carefully, for the purpose of covering the box, lest some one might happen to pass that way and get whatever there might be remaining in it. After covering it, he turned round to take the Record again, but behold it was gone, and where he knew not, neither did he know the means by which it had been taken from him.

At this, as a natural consequence, he was much alarmed. He kneeled down and asked the Lord why the Record had been taken from him; upon which the angel of the Lord appeared to him, and told him that he had not done as he had been commanded, for in a former revelation he had been commanded not to lay the plates down, or put them for a moment out of his hands, until he got into the house and deposited them in a chest or trunk, having a good lock and key, and, contrary to this, he had laid them down with the view of securing some fancied or imaginary treasure that remained.

In the moment of excitement, Joseph was overcome by the powers of darkness, and forgot the injunction that was laid upon him.

Having some further conversation with the angel on this occasion, Joseph was permitted to raise the stone again, when he beheld the plates as he had done before. He immediately reached forth his hand to take them, but instead of getting them, as he anticipated, he was hurled back upon the ground with great violence. When he recovered, the angel was gone, and he arose and returned to the house, weeping for grief and disappointment. (35)

What sort of additional "fancied or imaginary treasure," one may ask, could Joseph have been seeking when he laid down the plates in this version of the story? Why did he know "that probably there was something else in the box besides the plates"? What could conceivably have been of greater value than the Record itself? Of greater value than the marvelous history of the Mound-builders? Of greater value than the work so dear that the profits of its publication could place his family "*on a level* above the gener-ality of mankind"? Of such value that he would perform the forbid-den act of unhanding the plates to seek it out? Of such value that his very searching for it under the influence of the "powers of darkness" would cause its jealous guardian (an angel, in this ver-sion) to punish him by making the Record unavailable to him? He already knew of the breastplate and the magic translating stones (the "Urim" and "Thummim," as he would call them nine years later in ascribing to them a biblical origin). What else could there be? There is indeed an answer to these questions—one that will al-low a fuller exploration of the sexually based theme, but this pre-sumptive solution will have to wait until Chapter 7, after more background threads are woven into this tapestry of Joseph's fantasy.

Joseph's ongoing tale of the successive annual September 22 events from 1823 to 1827 is that of experimentation with a series of covisitors to the treasure site, as it appeared that just the right companion would be necessary to "consummate" the act of ob-taining the plates. Each of these individuals, Joseph apparently hoped and imagined, would act as the key that in some way would pacify the powerful paternal guardian of the treasure and so un-lock and overcome the latter's resistance to releasing it. As has al-ready been seen in the later narrations of the story, Alvin was the first to be named by this guardian, but Alvin's untimely death would serve as a puzzling obstacle that the young and clever hero would evidently have to surmount. Again, in Willard Chase's ret-rospective description:

> Joseph went one year from that day, to demand the book, and the spirit enquired for his brother, and he said that he was dead. The spirit then commanded him to come again, in just one year, and bring a man with him. On asking who might be the man, he was answered that he would know when he saw him.
>
> Joseph believed that one Samuel F. Lawrence [a fellow money-digger] was the man alluded to by the spirit, and went with him to a singular looking hill, in Manchester [near Palmyra, New York], and shewed him where the treasure was. Lawrence asked him if he had ever discovered anything with the plates of gold; he said no: he then asked

him to look in his stone, to see if there was anything with
them. He looked . . . and soon saw a pair of spectacles,
the same with which Joseph says he translated the Book
of Mormon . . . Not long after this, Joseph altered his mind,
and said L. was not the right man, nor had he told him the
right place. About this time he went to Harmony in Pennsylvania, and formed an acquaintance with a young lady, by the
name of Emma Hale, who he wished to marry. (36)

Again, it will be noted that the interest is focused not exclusively
on the plates, but on whether "there was anything with them."
     Another version of the story was related by Joseph, Jr. himself
to Emma's cousins Joseph and Hiel Lewis:

He [Joseph, Jr.] said that by a dream he was informed that at
such a place in a certain hill, in an iron box, were some gold
plates with curious engravings, which he must get and
translate, and write a book; that the plates were to be kept
concealed from every human being for a certain time, some
two or three years; that he went to the place and dug till he
came to the stone that covered the box, when he was
knocked down; that he again attempted to remove the
stone, and was again knocked down; this attempt was made
the third time, and the third time he was knocked down.
Then he exclaimed, "Why can't I get it?" or words to that effect; and then he saw a man standing over the spot, which to
him appeared like a Spaniard, having a long beard down
over his breast to about here, (Smith putting his hand to the
pit of his stomach) with his (the ghost's) throat cut from ear
to ear, and the blood streaming down, who told him that he
could not get it alone; that another person whom he, Smith,
would know at first sight, must come with him, and then he
would get it. And when Smith saw Miss Emma Hale, he
knew that she was the person . . .
     In all this narrative, there was not one word about "visions
of God," or of angels, or heavenly revelations. All his information was by that dream, and that bleeding ghost. (37)

Is it possible that the bleeding ghost in this version of the story
represents a familiar disguise? A decapitation fantasy is usually

a representation of castration in dream imagery, as the guardian ghost's neck in this scene is described as having been nearly cut through. And again, as in the Dogberry narrative quoted earlier in this chapter, the long beard could possibly represent the large phallus of the father-figure in the story, with the slash in the neck at its point of origin. If this is so, Joseph's gruesome fantasy then presents a nearly castrated father in the role of treasure guardian. It will be recalled that children who have faced terror at surgical operations typically have vivid fantasies in which they themselves wield the blade against the surgeon and the father, again reversing the roles of the dreadful event. But Joseph will never actually consummate the act in fantasy to kill his father directly. Such a thought, even in his dissociated world, was always to be an intolerable act, as in the original oedipal dilemma out of which the fantasy presumably arises.

With the introduction of Emma Hale, the story has now become capable of resolution through sexual consummation. Only a sexual key, through this interpretation, could unlock the prohibition of the paternal guardian of the treasure on the hill. If Joseph were to so present himself, the paternal adversary in his fantasy would no longer be able to protect his prize against the young rival. One might even suggest that Joseph's frightening conflict with Isaac Hale was woven into the treasure-seeking story through its reinforcement of the tyrannical father image of the treasure's guardian. On September 22, 1827, Emma accompanied Joseph up Hill Cumorah with a borrowed horse and wagon as he "obtained" the plates. Emma never saw them, nor, in the absence of angels, did anyone else.

Since *The Book of Mormon* is unquestionably a religious book, it should be expected to contain religious thematic material. However, there has been little to this point in the story of what in the Western tradition would usually pass for religion. It is indeed true that Joseph Smith, Jr. would write a religious book and attribute it to his translation of those plates he claimed to have found in a stone box on Hill Cumorah. To discover how this religious theme became the framework over which Joseph draped his sublimated fantasies, another digression needs to be made.

This digression leads back to Dartmouth College in Hanover, New Hampshire, six miles north of Joseph's fateful boyhood home in Lebanon. Dr. Nathan Smith, the doctor who performed surgery on young Joseph Smith, Jr., taught his medical students in a room at the north end of Dartmouth Hall, still a central edifice of the campus. Through the west windows of that room he could look a few yards away to the site of Old College Hall, where his colleague Professor John Smith taught. However, whereas Nathan was a brilliant and dynamic teacher, John was the paradigm of the absent-minded professor and the butt of many whispered campus jokes. Nevertheless, as professor of learned languages and the author of grammar textbooks in Greek, Latin, Hebrew, and Chaldean, John Smith possessed an organized and serious intellect with genuine curiosity. He was for many years a professor of religion and served as pastor of the Congregational Church on the Dartmouth campus. As a compulsive individual, he wrote out in advance all of his class lectures and sermons in a flourishing longhand, and many such manuscripts have survived. His religion class lectures, for instance, included a lengthy and detailed account of the destruction of Jerusalem by the Romans in 70 A.D.

One of the classes Professor John Smith taught at Dartmouth was "Natural Philosophy." All students took the course as part of the rigid curriculum of the time. In his surviving class notes of this series of lectures can be seen his descriptions of the wonders of astronomy, basic physics of air pressure, and the like. But the final lecture in this series was a grand departure from the physical subject matter of all that preceded it. After a short flowery introduction, he addressed a popular and controversial subject of his times by stating the following:

> Several opinions have been advanced by the learned, with respect to the first peopling of America.
>
> Some have thought the aboriginal natives of America do not escend from the sons of Noah, as the rest of mankind did. . . .
>
> The opinion that our Indians did not descend from the sons

of Noah is now, and deservedly universally discarded.

It is almost certain the aboriginal inhabitants of America are not the descendants of Jews, Christians, or Mahometans, because no trace of their religions have ever been found among them; nor had they ever heard the name of Moses, Christ, or Mahomet, till they were acquainted with the Europeans . . .

As the Carthaginians . . . were very early expert in sailing, and had frequent occasion to visit the Canary and Cape Verd[e] islands, it is not improbable that South America was peopled by them. The Carthaginian ships carried sometimes a thousand people, and were crowded with men, women and children, when they sent colonies to those islands; and doubtless, as they had not the advantage of the mariner's compass, some of them missed those islands, and were driven beyond their intended points. If this ever happened, they must of necessity be carried to America, which (part of South America I mean) lies but three weeks sail to the westward of the Canary and Cape Verd[e] islands. Without the use of this compass, it would be impossible for them to return to the eastern continent, on account of the trade winds being always opposite to them . . .[2]

Before I conclude this letter, I would just observe that it is probable China joins to the Continent of America. If this is the case, we may suppose that some of our Indian tribes came from that part of the world.

> I am, my dear Class
> with tenderest affection,
> your cordial friend
> and humble Ser[t]
> J Smith (38)

---

[2] Students of Mormon history will recognize in this paragraph a scenario similar to a story written by Solomon Spaulding, a Dartmouth graduate of the class of 1785. For many years, rumors had circulated that *The Book of Mormon* had been plagiarized from a lost manuscript of Spaulding's about ancient travelers to America. While such a manuscript was indeed found, it seems to bear more similarity to the above paragraph than to *The Book of Mormon*. This lecture of Professor John Smith's would have been heard by Spaulding in 1784 and could conceivably have planted the seed out of which Spaulding's fanciful story sprang.

Sitting in the classroom and listening to this lecture in 1789 was a young student, Ethan Smith, who would be graduated the following year. Upon leaving Dartmouth, Ethan founded and built the First Congregational Church in nearby Haverhill, New Hampshire, and served as its first pastor for nine years before moving to Hopkinton, New Hampshire and thence to the pastorate of the Congregational Church in Poultney, Vermont, about 1820. While in Poultney in 1823 he wrote and published the most unusual of his several religious books. This volume, *View of the Hebrews; or the Ten Tribes of Israel in America* (39), instantly became a very popular volume across New England and the frontier. The first edition sold out quickly, and a second edition with revisions was published in 1825 (40).

The thesis of *View of the Hebrews* was that the American Indians were descended from the lost ten tribes of Israel. Taking his cue from the eighteenth chapter of Isaiah, Ethan related his certainty that the "land shadowing with wings" where the lost tribes would be scattered was in reality the silhouetted continents of North and South America spreading like the wings of an eagle from the Panamanian peninsula. In his Congregationalist fervor, Ethan preached in his book that the mission of the American Christian community must be to bring the Indians back to their true heritage by educating them of their birthright and thus to bring about the "gathering of Israel," which would, in turn, usher in the millennium. Ethan Smith's theological notions carried a missionary zeal toward the Indians that paralleled the tradition of his alma mater.

Against the negative evidence for the Indians' Hebraic origins propounded by his former professor John Smith, Ethan argued, "If the Indians are of the tribes of Israel, some decisive evidence of this fact will ere long be exhibited" (41). Ethan's basic theory of the degradation of lofty Hebrew to primitive Indian culture was summarized well in his 1825 second edition:

> The probability then is this; that the ten tribes, arriving in this continent with some knowledge of the arts of civilized life; finding themselves in a vast wilderness filled with the best of game, inviting them to the chase; most of them fell

into a wandering idle hunting life. . . . More sensible parts of
these people associated together, to improve their knowledge of the arts; and probably continued thus for ages. From
these the noted relics of civilization discovered in the west
and south were furnished. But savage tribes prevailed; and
in process of time their savage jealousies and rage annihi-
lated their more civilized brethren. . . . This accounts for
their loss of the knowledge of letters, of the art of naviga-
tion, and the use of iron. (42)

This scenario is, of course, exactly the plotline elaborated by
Joseph Smith two to four years later throughout the nearly 600
pages of *The Book of Mormon.*

In further allegorical speculation about possible bits of evidence in support of his theory, Ethan Smith, in his first edition,
goes on to say:

The evidence discovered among the various tribes of Indians, of the truth of their Hebrew extraction, and of the divinity of their Old Testament, seems almost like finding, in the
various regions of America, various scrapes of an ancient Hebrew Old Testament . . . (43)

But as David Persuitte points out (44), Ethan, in the second edition of his book, substitutes the following for the above paragraph:

Some readers have said; if the Indians are of the tribes of
Israel, some decisive evidence of the fact will ere long be exhibited. Suppose a leading character in Israel—wherever
they are—should be found to have had in possession some
biblical fragment of ancient Hebrew writing. This man dies,
and it is buried with him in such a manner as to be long pre-
served. Some people afterwards removing that earth, discover this fragment, and ascertain what it is—an article of
ancient Israel. (45)

Ethan developed this line of speculation even further in a tan-
talizing way. He discussed rumors of discovery of Hebrew-lettered
parchment fragments that were subsequently lost. He discussed

a tale told by an old Indian that his ancestors had had an old book which they had long since lost the ability to read, so they buried it with an Indian chief. And finally in the appendix of the second edition of his book, Ethan wrote about a criticism made of his first edition:

> . . . Moses . . . was inspired to write the book of God. . . . Now was there during all this time, in the other nations of the east, the knowledge of *another book of God* . . . that the descendants of the northern barbarous nations might bring down many deep and correct impressions of it . . . in so distant and extensive a region of the world as this continent? (46)

This lost-book hypothesis was all Joseph needed to add the final dimension to his story of the Moundbuilders. The fantasies arising through his dissociations had tormented him since the age of seven. Thanks to the archaeological speculations in his local newspapers, he had already begun to frame these fantasies around an imaginary culture of the Moundbuilders buried in his neighborhood. As a teenager Joseph had repeatedly recited this combination of elements to his family around the evening fireplace. Now Ethan Smith would hand him the final dimension that would increase the importance of his work by several orders of magnitude. As though building an Indian tepee, Joseph would lash together the solid pillars of Ethan's book into a rigid frame and drape the buffalo hides of his dissociated fantasies over it to create an imposing unified structure—something so impressive and different from its component parts that neither could be recognized. The angry, threatening, and jealous apparitions springing from the dissociated part of his mind would become ancient Hebrews. They would escape chaos in their world by banishing themselves to the seashore (as Joseph had been so banished after his childhood operations) and building boats to sail to America (perhaps dramatizing for Joseph a frequent childhood fantasy—"I'll show them. I'll sail away and never come back. Then they'll be sorry.") His characters would act out their vengeful vignettes against one another on the stage of the American continents. These subplots would follow Ethan Smith's grand scheme wherein savagery would eventually triumph over civilization. However, throughout would be the domination by the invincible hero—what Freud called "His Majesty the Ego" (47)—transfiguring phoenix-like from generation to generation, wielding the great knife himself, and winning battle after battle against persecuting evil forces on all sides. Over and over, betrayal, patricide, and dismemberment would substitute in a colorful variety of disguises for a horrifying, real-world event of the author's own childhood bedroom. And finally, interwoven throughout the text of fantasy would be many self-aggrandizing predictions of the future translation of the book itself by its prophetic author Joseph, whose father would bear the same name.

But Ethan Smith's book alone probably would not have been sufficient to have given Joseph the zeal to pursue a religious basis for his emerging project. There had also been in his teenage environment a powerful evangelical movement. The tent meetings, hellfire-breathing preachers, and crazed, born-again revivalist converts were a major part of the social scene of upstate New York in the 1820s. The region had gained the nickname the "burnt-over district," as Methodist, Presbyterian, and other sectarian Pentecostal movements had swept across the area, with sinners being exhorted to save themselves from Satan's temptations. If his intense ambivalence toward fatherlike persons was a reality, Joseph could scarcely have avoided developing troubling inner feelings toward these austere, guilt-inspiring men. Joseph was described by an acquaintance as having caught "a spark of Methodism in the camp meeting, away down in the woods, on the Vienna road, [and] he was a very passable exhorter in the evening meetings" (48). However, because Alvin's death in 1823 had been very troubling for Joseph, he sought baptism and affiliation with the local Baptist Church that year during one of the greatest revivals (49). Furthermore, Joseph would later attempt to join the Harmony [Pennsylvania] Methodist Episcopal Church in 1828 after another death in the family, but would be refused membership because, as the church leaders decided,

> such a character as he was a disgrace to the church, that he
> could not be a member of the church unless he broke off his

sins by repentance, made public confession, renounced his
fraudulent and hypocritical practices, and gave some evidence that he intended to reform and conduct himself
somewhat nearer like a christian than he had done. (50)

Joseph would immediately withdraw his name from considera-
tion for membership on that occasion, having been on the rolls
only three days.

But Joseph's identification with the several charismatic revivalist preachers he had encountered would have been expected to
be intense. Despite his later resentful exhortations against
"priest-craft," he might well have experienced considerable envy
of these powerful figures, with their rhetorical abilities to gain
emotional supremacy over their cowering subjects. If something
inside him did, indeed, regard itself as God, he would surely have
to be able to demonstrate skills at least commensurate with these
powerful rivals. Compared with them, his own charismatic
achievements with farmers in cornfields must have looked humble indeed.

The earliest record of a religious essence involving the gold
plates (other than the much later retrospective accounts by Joseph and his mother) appears in the fall of 1827 in connection
with the financing of the writing. Specifically, Joseph had occasionally worked for a well-to-do farmer named Martin Harris, who
was intensely interested in religious matters and who had reportedly passed through a denominational odyssey as Quaker, Univer-
salist, Restorationist, Baptist, and Presbyterian. Joseph persuaded
his mother to visit Harris, to tell the farmer about the discovery of
the plates, and to invite him over for a visit. Harris later related the
visit with Joseph as follows:

> I took him by the arm and led him away from the rest, and
> requested him to tell me the story, which he did as follows,
> He said: "An angel had appeared to him, and told him it was
> God's work." . . . Joseph had before this described the man-
> ner of his finding the plates. He found them by looking in
> the stone found in the well of Mason Chase. The family had
> likewise told me the same thing.
>   Joseph said the angel told him he must quit the company

of the money-diggers. That there were wicked men among
them. He must have no more to do with them. He must not
lie, nor swear, nor steal. He told him to go and look in the
spectacles, and he would show him the man that would assist him. That he did so, and saw myself, Martin Harris,
standing before him. That struck me with surprise. I told
him I wished him to be very careful about these things.
"Well," said he, "I saw you standing before me as plainly as I
do now." I said, if it is the devil's work I will have nothing to
do with it; but if it is the Lord's you can have all the money
necessary to bring it before the world. . . . Now you must
not blame me for not taking your word. If the Lord will
show me that it is his work, you can have all the money you
want. (51)

Since Harris's passion for religion seemed to parallel his passion for financial success, the project was doubly appealing. As
the Reverend John Clark said of Harris after the latter had summarized his meeting with Joseph:

The whole thing appeared to me so ludicrous and purile,
that I could not refrain from telling Mr. Harris, that I believed it a mere hoax got up to practice upon his credulity, or
an artifice to extort from him money; for I had already, in the
course of the conversation, learned that he had advanced
some twenty-five dollars to Jo Smith as a sort of premium for
sharing with him in the glories and profits of this new revelation. For at this time, his mind seemed to be quite as intent
upon the pecuniary advantage that would arise from the
possession of the plates of solid gold of which this book was
composed, as upon the spiritual light it would diffuse over
the world. (52)

Harris' wife Lucy was yet more skeptical and harbored a
strong fear that her husband's involvement with Joseph would
bring them to financial ruin:

Martin Harris was once industrious, attentive to his domes-
tic concerns, and thought to be worth about ten thousand
dollars. . . . About a year previous to the report being raised
that Smith had found gold plates, he became very intimate

> with the Smith family, and said he believed Joseph could see
> in his stone anything he wished . . .
>   . . . His whole object was to make money by it. . . . One
> day, while at Peter Harris' house, I told him he had better
> leave the company of the Smiths as their religion was false;
> to which he replied, if you would let me alone, I could make
> money by it. (53)

Joseph, in the meantime, was beginning to feel the resentment from his fellow money-digging companions who felt that if
the young glass-looker had indeed found any gold plates, they
should rightfully be the property of the entire group. But because
Joseph seemed to have been driven more by his own deep-seated
conflicts than by peer pressures, he turned his back on his former
companions and returned to the Hale farm in Harmony, Pennsylvania, with a heavy wooden box in the wagon. Then, as the hap-
less and frustrated Isaac Hale related,

> Soon after this, I was informed they had brought a wonder-
> ful book of Plates down with them. I was shown a box in
> which it is said they were contained, which had to all ap-
> pearances, been used as a glass box of the common window
> glass. I was allowed to feel the weight of the box, and they
> gave me to understand that the book of plates was then in
> the box—into which, however, I was not allowed to look.
>   I inquired of Joseph Smith Jr., who was to be the first who
> would be allowed to see the Book of Plates? He said it was a
> young child. After this, I became dissatisfied, and informed
> him that if there was anything in my house of that descrip-
> tion, which I could not be allowed to see, he must take it
> away; if he did not, I was determined to see it. After that, the
> Plates were said to be hid in the woods. (54)

There were other accounts as well in which Joseph had said
that the first person to see the plates would be a young child.
Since Emma was pregnant at the time and would deliver their
child nine to ten months after the "acquisition" of the plates, this
reference seems to be further confirmation of the sexual symbolism surrounding Joseph's possession of the treasure. This might
suggest further that he was already beginning to develop unusual

identification with his unborn child. In Chapter 6 it will become clear that this child would play an additional role for Joseph.

Even though the plates were supposedly hidden in the woods, Joseph began to "translate" them by one or more of his magic spectacles or seer-stones. Because he lacked literacy skills, he would dictate his phrases to Emma, who would, in turn, transcribe them. It has been speculated by Brodie and others that this early portion of the book contained enough religious flavor to satisfy Martin Harris but was otherwise a fairly secular history of the Moundbuilders (55).

It is a fair assumption that the act of translation was the product, at least in part, of utterances made in trancelike states. Indeed, Emma's own descriptions appear to support this:

> I frequently wrote day after day, often sitting at the table close by him, he sitting with his face buried in his hat with the stone in it and dictating hour after hour. (56)

> One time while he was translating he stopped suddenly, *pale as a sheet,* and said, "Emma, did Jerusalem have walls around it?" When I answered, "Yes," he replied "Oh! I was afraid I had been deceived." (57) (emphasis added)

Harris came to visit the young couple in their poverty in February 1828, and Joseph, probably wishing to impress his patron, gave him a sheet of paper with some "reformed Egyptian" characters on it that, Joseph stated, he had copied from the plates.[3] Harris promptly took the paper overland to New York City, where he gained an audience with Professor Charles Anthon, professor of Greek and Latin at Columbia University. Anthon's own account of the visit is as follows:

> The whole story about my having pronounced the Mormonite inscription to be "reformed Egyptian hieroglyphics"

---

[3] One wonders, in view of his newly pregnant wife, his new prospects for a fresh start at prosperity, and the abandonment of his money-digging companions, if Joseph's choice of the adjective "reformed" at this time might have applied semiconsciously to himself as much as to the characters on the plates.

is *perfectly false.* Some years ago, a plain, and apparently simple-hearted farmer, called upon me with a note from Dr. Mitchell of our city, now deceased, requesting me to decypher, if possible, a paper, which the farmer would hand me, and which Dr. M. confessed he had been unable to understand. Upon examining the paper in question, I soon came to the conclusion that it was all a trick, perhaps a *hoax.* When I asked the person, who brought it, how he obtained the writing, he gave me . . . the following account: A "gold book," . . . had been dug up in the northern part of the state of New York, and along with the book an enormous pair of "*gold spectacles*"! . . . Whoever examined the plates through the spectacles, was enabled not only to *read* them, but fully to *understand* their meaning. All this knowledge, however, was confined at that time to a young man, who had the trunk containing the book and spectacles in his sole possession. This young man was placed behind a curtain, . . . and, thus concealed from view, . . . decyphered the characters of the book. . . . Not a word, however, was said about the plates having been decyphered "by the gift of God." . . . The farmer added, that he had been requested to contribute a sum of money towards the publication of the "golden book." . . . As a last precautionary step, however, he had resolved to come to New York, and obtain the opinion of the learned about the meaning of the paper which he brought with him, and which had been given him as a part of the contents of the book, although no translation had been furnished at the time by the young man with the spectacles. On hearing this odd story, I . . . began to regard it as a part of a scheme to cheat the farmer of his money, and I communicated my suspicions to him. . . . This paper was in fact a singular scrawl. It consisted of all kinds of crooked characters in columns, and had evidently been prepared by some person who had before him at the time a book containing various alphabets. Greek and Hebrew letters, crosses and flourishes, Roman letters inverted or placed sideways, were arranged in perpendicular columns, and the whole ended in a rude delineation of a circle divided into various compartments, decked with various strange marks, and evidently copied after the Mexican Calender [*sic*] given by Humboldt, but copied in such a way as not to betray the source whence

it was derived. . . . I . . . well remember that the paper contained anything but *"Egyptian Hieroglyphics."* (58)

In fact, it has been pointed out that when that surviving page of
characters is inverted, the names JOS and JOE may be clearly recognized amidst the various symbols. Subsequent contemporary
analyses have shown no resemblance between the characters and
Egyptian or any other known ancient script.

Harris returned to Harmony in April 1828, still trusting in the
project, and took over the transcription duties from Emma. Joseph
would hang a blanket between the two of them so that Harris could
not see him while he dictated. But with the plates ostensibly hidden in the woods, where Joseph claimed he could see them with
his face buried in his hat and looking into his stone, the reason for
the blanket is obscure, although it has has been speculated that Joseph might have been from time to time using other reference materials for assistance. Joseph warned Harris that if he should peek
behind the blanket, God's wrath would strike him down.

By June, 116 manuscript pages were complete, or about one
page per day since the process had begun. With the baby due any
day, bringing a likely break in the literary process, Joseph consented to let Harris take the manuscript back to his skeptical wife
to prove to her that the project was indeed worthwhile. Under any
other circumstances, Joseph would almost certainly have declined such a request because of his enormous personal investment in his project, to say nothing of his sense of persecution by
others and the obvious possibility of theft of the manuscript. But
the immediate prospect of the arrival of a child—of an extension
of himself—must surely have overridden all other considerations
at that time.

Two tragedies struck almost at once. The infant lived only
three hours and was "very much deformed" (59), with Emma
nearly dying during delivery. Both the child's death and Emma's
condition were very possibly the result of the malnutrition she
likely suffered in their poverty. Then the manuscript disappeared.
On his trip back to Palmyra in search of his manuscript once
Emma had recovered some strength, Joseph was met by an abject
Martin and a triumphant Lucy Harris, the latter of whom had hid-

den (or destroyed) the manuscript and who tauntingly defied him
to translate the pages verbatim again.

Joseph was plunged into that awful abyss of emotional numb-
ness wherein he was unable to mourn for two catastrophic losses
at once, either of which alone would have been crippling. It was
immediately after the death of his newborn that, as noted earlier
in this chapter, he sought membership in the local Methodist
Church and was so humiliatingly rebuffed by the church "fathers."

In his bitter solitude Joseph faced the stark realities of his
losses. He could not make another attempt at redictating the
same material because his inability to reproduce it word-for-word
would, if the former 116 pages still existed, set up a possible challenge to his "gift." If he could not continue translating, Emma
might no longer believe in his "gift" either, and on this so much of
his perception of their relationship undoubtedly rested. If he
could not resolve his dilemma, he would lose the financial support of Martin Harris, seemingly the only source of income he
had. He would be mercilessly humiliated by his father-in-law. And,
finally, his own original family, counting on the proceeds from his
book sales to prevent foreclosure on their farm, would lose everything unless he could find a solution (60).

But even more threatening than these substantial threats in
the world of reality were the troubling fantasies undoubtedly
bubbling up in vague form from the dissociated recesses of his
mind. Was his grotesquely deformed child in some way a symbol
of the crippling of his manhood? Was he in some way irreparably
impaired because of that horror-filled punishment of his childhood? And what of his treasure? Was its "theft" a further mockery
of the forbidden triumph he had experienced in its acquisition?
Was he being victimized again in a further repetition of his earlier
trauma? As both losses seem to have had profound sexual significance in his unconscious, they should have produced a most intense conflict.

The overwhelming sense of powerlessness engendered by the
punishment of his double loss must have strained all of Joseph's
coping mechanisms to the breaking point, especially after his humiliating rejection by the one outside resource, the Methodist
Church, to which he had turned for support. His torment and

humiliation had become unbearable. Now, for the first time, in July 1828, he received a direct reprimand from God. Joseph began to hear voices speaking aloud to him. If he had had to suffer this badly in life, it must be (as before in childhood) that he had deserved to be punished; and some mighty representation of his father deep in his own mind must again do the chastising, as at the age of seven. Far down in the black market of Joseph's psyche, shadowy presences had bartered the deadly hemlock of shame for the hallucinogenic mushrooms of guilt. It was the only way.

What had he done to incur all of this wrath? As in his childhood bedroom, whatever fantasies existed in his own world of guilt must, by definition, be the source of the problem. After all, it was just ten months before that he had acted out a sexually significant ritual in the acquisition of a treasure. Performance of this ritual had coincided with the conception of a child. Now precisely the same kind of action for which he fantasized that he was so painfully punished in childhood was being repeated again. But this time in Joseph's fantasy the father-presence punished him by making a mockery of that sexuality—by hideously deforming his dead infant and by taking away the pleasurable fruit of his treasure quest. Joseph's sexuality was unbreakably linked with the threat of violence. His chastising revelation from the God within confirmed the link:

> The works, and the designs, and the purposes of God cannot be frustrated, neither can they come to nought, . . .

> For although a man may have many revelations, and have power to do many mighty works, yet if he boasts in his own strength, and sets at nought the counsels of God, and *follows after the dictates of his own will and carnal desires, he must fall and incur the vengeance of a just God upon him.* . . .

> And behold, how oft you have transgressed the commandments and the laws of God, and have gone on in the persuasions of men; . . .

> Yet you should have been faithful and *he would have extended his arm and supported you against all the fiery*

darts of the adversary [Dr. Nathan Smith's, perhaps?]; and he would have been with you in every time of trouble. . . .

Behold, thou art Joseph, and thou wast chosen to do the work of the Lord, but because of transgression, if thou art not aware thou wilt fall; . . .

But remember God is merciful; therefore, repent of that which thou hast done which is contrary to the command- ment which I gave you, and thou art still chosen, and art again called to the work; . . .

Except thou do this, thou shalt be delivered up and become as other men, and have no more gift. (61) (emphasis added)

But in the same way that he "atoned" for his fantasized sexual sins in childhood (which, as noted in Chapter 3, is a common pro- cess in children immobilized by illness or injury) by undergoing the torment of his operations and their aftermath, did Joseph now feel again a semblance of atonement through having suffered these double losses of adulthood? In this unstable but driven frame of mind he set out anew to assuage his inner troubles by narrating *The Book of Mormon.*

Joseph's dictation was more facile the second time and was ac- companied by considerable support from his parents. The prob- lem of the 116 pages was dealt with by telling the story from a different vantage point so that, if found, the pages would not in- validate the claim of divinity of what constituted the final book. Regardless of the content of the original work, the story now be- came a grand and violent religious morality play in which right- eousness prevailed and evil was destroyed.

The pace quickened to a frenzy with the arrival in April 1829 of Oliver Cowdery, a young schoolteacher, who would board with the Smith family and serve as Joseph's transcriptionist. The Cowdery family had lived in Poultney, Vermont, and had been members of Ethan Smith's Congregational pastorate. Oliver had left Poultney in 1825, the year the second edition of *View of the Hebrews* was pub- lished. He must have known of its message explicitly. Furthermore, Oliver's father had been involved as one of the "rodsmen" in the Wood Scrape affair in 1802 (see Chapter 2), and Oliver himself was reported to have a gift with the divining rod, a fact that impressed Joseph very much. Oliver was the perfect collaborator.

The manuscript of the *Book of Mormon* arrived at the printer in 1829, virtually without punctuation marks and with lamentable grammar and endless run-on sentences. Martin Harris, by this time divorced from his wife, had had to sell his farm to finance the book's publication. Lucy Harris's prescience had allowed her to escape with the security of eighty acres and a house free of encumbrance. On March 26, 1830, the book went on sale in the Palmyra bookstore.

Notes

1. Fraiberg S: "Tales of the Discovery of the Secret Treasure." *Psychoanalytic Study of the Child* 9:218–241, 1954; see p. 218.
2. Ibid., p. 239.
3. Ibid., p. 241.
4. Brodie F: *No Man Knows My History: The Life of Joseph Smith, the Mormon Prophet,* 2nd Edition. New York, Alfred A. Knopf, 1989, p. 19.
5. Purple WD: "Reminiscence, 28 APR 1877." See also Quinn M: *Early Mormonism and the Magic World View.* Salt Lake City, Signature Books, 1987, p. 39.
6. Capron J: "Affidavit," in Howe ED: *Mormonism Unvailed.* Painesville, OH, 1834, p. 259.
7. Stafford W: "Affidavit," in Howe ED: *Mormonism Unvailed,* p. 239.
8. Hale I: "Affidavit," in Howe ED: *Mormonism Unvailed,* p. 263.
9. *Laws of the State of New York Revised and Passed . . . ,* revisors Van Ness WP, Woodworth J. See also Persuitte D: *Joseph Smith and the Origins of The Book of Mormon.* Jefferson, NC, McFarland & Company, 1985, p. 54.
10. Record of the trial of Joseph Smith for disorderly conduct, Bainbridge, NY, March 20, 1826. Published in the *New Schaff–Herzog Encyclopedia of Religious Knowledge,* Vol. 2. New York, 1883, p. 1576. See also Brodie F: *No Man Knows My History,* 2nd Edition, pp. 427–428.

11. Record of the trial of Joseph Smith for disorderly conduct, Bainbridge, NY, March 20, 1826.

12. Ibid.

13. Ibid.

14. Noble JK: Letter to J. B. Turner, March 8, 1842. See also Persuitte D: *Joseph Smith and the Origins of The Book of Mormon,* p. 154.

15. Hale I: "Affidavit," p. 263.

16. Ingersoll P: "Affidavit," in Howe ED: *Mormonism Unvailed,* pp. 234–235.

17. Briggs EC, Peterson JW: Interview with Smith W. *Deseret News* [Salt Lake City], January 20, 1894. See also Brodie F: *No Man Knows My History,* 2nd Edition, pp. 27–28.

18. Smith J Sr: *Wayne (NY) Sentinel,* September 25, 1824. Quoted in Brodie F: *No Man Knows My History,* 2nd Edition, p. 28.

19. Smith LM: *Biographical Sketches of Joseph Smith the Prophet and His Progenitors for Many Generations.* Liverpool, S. W. Richards, 1853 [reprinted New York, Arno Press, 1969], p. 85.

20. Quoted in Brodie F: *No Man Knows My History,* 2nd Edition, p. 34.

21. Cited in Brodie F: *No Man Knows My History,* 2nd Edition, p. 35.

22. *Palmyra (NY) Herald,* February 19, 1823. Quoted in Brodie F: *No Man Knows My History,* 2nd Edition, p. 34.

23. Chase P: "Affidavit," in Howe ED: *Mormonism Unvailed,* p. 248.

24. Dogberry O: *Palmyra (NY) Reflector,* February 14, 1831, Article Number IV. Quoted in Brodie F: *No Man Knows My History,* 2nd Edition, p. 430.

25. Capron J: "Affidavit," in Howe ED: *Mormonism Unvailed,* p. 260.

26. Smith J: *Manuscript History of the Church,* Book A-1. Salt Lake City, LDS Church Archives. Quoted in Vogel D (ed): *Early Mormon Documents,* Vol. 1. Salt Lake City, Signature Books, 1996, p. 67.

27. Freud S: *The Interpretation of Dreams* (1900). Translated and edited by Brill AA. New York, Macmillan Co., 1913, pp. 130–131.

28. Copley L: "Testimony," in Howe ED: *Mormonism Unvailed,* pp. 276–277.
29. Green J: *Slang Through the Ages.* Lincolnwood, IL, NTC Publishing Group, 1996, p. 50.
30. Smith J: *Manuscript History of the Church,* Book A-1. Salt Lake City, LDS Church Archives. Quoted in Vogel D (ed): *Early Mormon Documents,* Vol. 1. Salt Lake City, Signature Books, 1996, p. 67.
31. Ibid.
32. Chase W. "Affidavit," in Howe ED: *Mormonism Unvailed,* pp. 242–243.
33. Quinn M: *Early Mormonism and the Magic World View.* Salt Lake City, Signature Books, 1987, p. 132.
34. Bettelheim B: *The Uses of Enchantment: The Meaning and Importance of Fairy Tales.* New York, Vintage Books, 1975, pp. 289–291.
35. Smith LM: *Biographical Sketches of Joseph Smith the Prophet and His Progenitors for Many Generations,.* pp. 85–86.
36. Chase W: "Affidavit," in Howe ED: *Mormonism Unvailed,* pp. 242–243.
37. Lewis J, Lewis H: Letter, "Mormon History." *Amboy (IL) Journal,* April 30, 1879. Quoted in Persuitte D: *Joseph Smith and the Origins of The Book of Mormon,* pp. 73–74
38. Smith J[ohn]: Class lecture notes, Natural Philosophy (Lecture 12), January 1779. Baker Library Archives, Dartmouth College, Hanover, NH.
39. Smith E: *View of the Hebrews; or the Ten Tribes of Israel in America.* Poultney, VT, 1823.
40. Smith E: *View of the Hebrews; or the Ten Tribes of Israel in America,* 2nd Edition. Poultney, VT, 1825.
41. Ibid., p. 217.
42. Ibid., p. 172.
43. Smith E: *View of the Hebrews,* 1823, p. 167.
44. Persuitte D: *Joseph Smith and the Origins of The Book of Mormon,* p. 117.
45. Smith E: *View of the Hebrews,* 2nd Edition, p. 217.
46. Ibid., p. 280.

47. Freud S: "The Relationship of the Poet to Day-dreaming" (1908), in *Collected Papers,* Vol. 4. Translated and edited by Riviere J. New York, Basic Books, 1959, p. 173.

48. Turner O: *History of the Pioneer Settlement of Phelps and Gorham's Purchase,* p. 214. Quoted in Brodie F: *No Man Knows My History,* 2nd Edition, p. 26.

49. Lapham F: "The Mormons." *Historical Magazine,* Vol. 8, Second Ser., No. 5., May 1870, pp. 305–306. Cited in Persuitte D: *Joseph Smith and the Origins of The Book of Mormon,* p. 31.

50. Lewis J, Lewis H: Letter. *Amboy (IL) Journal,* April 30, 1879. See also Newell LK, Avery VT: *Mormon Enigma: Emma Hale Smith.* Garden City, NY, Doubleday & Co., 1984, p. 25.

51. Tiffany J: "Mormonism—No. II." *Tiffany's Monthly,* Vol. 5, No. 4, August 1859, pp. 168–169. Quoted in Persuitte D: *Joseph Smith and the Origins of The Book of Mormon,* p. 70.

52. Clark JA: *Gleanings by the Way.* New York, 1842, p. 224. See also Persuitte D: *Joseph Smith and the Origins of The Book of Mormon,* p. 71.

53. Harris L: "Affidavit," in Howe ED: *Mormonism Unvailed,* pp. 254–256.

54. Hale I: "Affidavit," in Howe ED: *Mormonism Unvailed,* p. 264.

55. See Brodie F: *No Man Knows My History,* pp. 55–56.

56. Smith J III: "Notes of Interview With Emma Smith Bidamon," February 1879, Miscellany, RLDS Church Library–Archives, Independence, MO.

57. Briggs EC: "A Visit to Nauvoo in 1856." *Journal of History* 9(January):454, 1916. Quoted in Vogel D (ed): *Early Mormon Documents,* Vol. 1. p. 530.

58. Anthon C: "Affidavit," in Howe ED: *Mormonism Unvailed,* pp. 270–272.

59. Lewis S: *Susquehanna Register,* May 1, 1834. Cited in Howe ED: *Mormonism Unvailed,* p. 269.

60. See Brodie F: *No Man Knows My History,* 2nd Edition, p. 55.

61. *Doctrine and Covenants,* Section 3, vv. 1, 4, 6, 8–11. Salt Lake City, Deseret News Company, 1880, pp. 81–82.

Trance-lation

*F*or those not acquainted with *The Book of Mormon,* a brief review of the plotline is in order. There are in the book two separate narratives of ancient Old World Hebraic families who encounter chaos in their lives in the Holy Land and escape to the seashore, where they build boats and travel across the ocean to the Americas. As their numbers expand, they develop advanced civilizations over the succeeding centuries, become involved in bloody wars, and ultimately kill each other off, the few savage survivors continuing as the contemporary American Indians.

One of the two families, the Jaredite group, leaves the Holy Land about 3000 B.C. as a result of the Old Testament incident of the building of the Tower of Babel, when the common language was confounded.[1]

The other family, under the patriarch Lehi, leaves for the Western Hemisphere about 600 B.C.

---

[1] To be precise, the Jaredites could not have been Hebraic because of their pre-Abrahamic existence, but this seems not to have troubled the author.

after receiving a premonition of the impending destruction of Jerusalem. The Jaredites completely annihilate themselves prior to the arrival of the family of Lehi.

Throughout *The Book of Mormon,* society demonstrates a distinctly bipolar structure. In the very large segment of the book devoted to the family and descendants of Lehi (the Jaredite story is told in the final 35 of the book's 590 pages), good and evil are starkly portrayed by racial designation. The patriarch Lehi has several sons, some of whom, like Nephi, are pure and righteous, but the remainder of which, like Laman, are evil and lazy. The latter are cursed early in the narrative by being changed from "white and exceedingly fair and delightsome" to dark and "loathsome." There are neither societal nor personal grays or tans in *The Book of Mormon.*

These two groups, the white "Nephites" and the dark "Lamanites," become the protagonists around which the many subplots of *The Book of Mormon* are woven. Sudden conversions from righteous to evil and the reverse occur frequently among individuals and groups of both races, but all characters are unidimensional at any one moment. Character development is usually limited to acceptance or rejection of religious orthodoxy. Action is commonly in the form of warfare and long sermonlike speeches threatening punishment for evildoing.

The repetitiveness of the plotline is interrupted only slightly by the physical arrival of Jesus Christ in the Americas immediately after the crucifixion in Jerusalem. This event ushers in a period of societal and individual perfection lasting exactly 200 years, following which the bipolar pattern again ensues. Thereafter, strife and battles become more massive in scale, until the Lamanites kill all of the Nephites except for one, Moroni, who completes the historical record of the Nephites and Lamanites, translates and transcribes the old records of the Jaredites onto metal plates, and buries all of them in Hill Cumorah, near Lake Ontario, in what will one day become New York State.

Several of Joseph Smith's biographers have suggested that certain aspects of *The Book of Mormon* appear to resemble material that was a part of its author's own environment and experience. Thus, the concept has developed that the book is an

amalgamation of overlapping themes of personal significance to
Joseph Smith, Jr. However, several less-than-obvious themes arising from his inner conflicts are probably of greater significance
than many of those already outlined.

Some of the themes apparently drawn from Ethan Smith's
View of the Hebrews have already been described in Chapter 4.
Among these is the mission of Anglo-Americans to convert the Indians to Christianity in the "latter days" and to bring them to
a knowledge of their Hebraic origins, thereby bringing about the
millennium. As Brodie points out (1), other themes include the
fact that both *View of the Hebrews* and *The Book of Mormon* begin
with reference to the destruction of Jerusalem,[2] tell of inspired
prophets among the ancient Americans, quote Old Testament
scripture (King James version) at length and almost exclusively
from Isaiah, and postulate that the ancient Americans had developed an advanced civilization. Ethan Smith describes "copper
breastplates" unearthed from Indian mounds to which were af-
fixed two white buckhorn buttons "in resemblance of the Urim
and Thummim." And finally, Ethan marvels at the story of Quetzal-
coatl, the bearded, white Aztec God whom the author describes as
"a type of Christ"; Joseph merely extends this metaphor by describing Christ himself coming to the Americas (2).

Persuitte (3) describes other instances in which thematic *The
Book of Mormon* material was apparently borrowed from *View of
the Hebrews.* Ethan Smith makes it plain that only nine-and-a-half
of the Ten Lost Tribes had been taken captive by the Assyrians,
with half of the tribe of Manasseh remaining free. In *The Book of
Mormon,* the patriarch of the family that escapes to the Americas
is described as "a descendent of Manasseh," presumably from the
remnant of the one tribe that remained free. Persuitte further describes, through scores of side-by-side comparisons, convincing
parallels between the two books in plotlines, proper names, and
religious messages.

A second thematic source of material seems to have arisen out

---

[2] It will be remembered that Dartmouth's Professor John Smith delivered
a memorable lecture on this subject to Ethan Smith's class.

of the bitter anti-Masonic movement that swept upstate New York in the late 1820s (4). This fervor seems to have had its origins in the mysterious murder in 1826 of William Morgan, a Mason who was then in the process of printing an exposé of Freemasonry. (As will be described in Chapter 7, Morgan's widow would later become one of Joseph's plural wives.) Many of the popular anti-Masonic phrases and perceptions appear to have been given life in *The Book of Mormon* in the form of the secret band of "Gadianton robbers" with their satanic rituals, murderous activities, and secret laws and oaths, all working to subvert the legitimate social order.

Several other minor sources of thematic material for *The Book of Mormon* seem to have arisen from various other corners of Joseph's social environment, including that of American patriotic lore. A reference to the "God of Nature" in I Nephi 5[3] is possibly a paraphrase from the first sentence of the United States Declaration of Independence. Frequent references to a "land of liberty" and to the undemocratic nature of rule by kings reflect a more American nationalist viewpoint than a Hebraic one. And it seems somehow appropriate that "King Lib" should have destroyed the plague of serpents and led his people to happiness and prosperity.

The American frontier makes its appearance in spirit and substance, for example, in the imagery of hearts hardening "like unto a flint." Over and over, heroes in *The Book of Mormon* escape into the refuge of the wilderness, where their lives are enriched by a fresh start. The idea of being "wanderers in a strange land" was quite a familiar concept to Joseph Smith's family and thousands like them in the America of the 1820s.

---

[3] All quotations from and citations to *The Book of Mormon* refer to the first edition (1830) in order to be as close to Joseph Smith, Jr.'s language and original intent as possible. The reader will therefore notice frequent grammatical and spelling errors in direct quotations from this book. The chapters in the first edition are identical in content (though revised in wording) to the chapters in the contemporary version in use by the Reorganized Church. The chapter delimitations in the contemporary version in use by the Utah-based Latter-Day Saints usually bear little relation to those in the first edition. A reproduction of the 1830 edition was published by Herald Publishing House, Independence, Missouri, in 1970.

It is possible that the epileptic seizures of Joseph's grandfather Mack make their appearance as well. In numerous instances evil individuals in *The Book of Mormon* are typically seen to "quake and fall to earth" as a form of punishment or retribution from God. The Lamanite king, Lamoni, in particular, was so evil that his postictal state lasted for three days. In each case the convulsions are given a mystical significance, perhaps a reflection of the powerful emotional impact that the witnessing of a grand mal seizure would have had on the author as a terrified child.

In the second edition of her biography of Joseph Smith, Brodie breaks important ground in dealing with thematic material in *The Book of Mormon.* In the supplement to that volume she begins to look for parallels between Joseph's family relationships and various patterns of behavior in the book. She suggests that sibling rivalry and fratricide are the principal themes, drawing the important parallel between Lehi and his six sons (four righteous and two evil), on the one hand, and Joseph Smith, Sr. and his six sons, on the other (each group of brothers sharing in common the two names Samuel and Joseph). Brodie also points out the extensive use in *The Book of Mormon* of the Old Testament story of Joseph, who was the subject of homicidal wishes by his brothers. (Siblings, according to Shengold, "tend to be the first scapegoats of the abused child" [5], whether in action or projected fantasy.) Brodie further suggests that the behavioral polarity seen in *The Book of Mormon* might represent both sides of conflicts existing in Joseph's own psyche: the dark world of black magic and money-digging versus the new white world of religion and Christian salvation. "Was he, in truth," she asks, "Lamanite or Nephite?" (6).

Brodie cites, in particular, the event in Joseph, Jr.'s life at the age of fourteen when, as described by his mother, "a gun was fired across his pathway, with the evident intention of shooting him" (7). After a thorough search, no perpetrator could be found. Brodie wonders if this incident caused Joseph to harbor fantasies that the attacker was one of his own brothers, since the event happened near the doorway of the family's home. Although this incident may indeed have had such an effect on Joseph, any such thoughts did not likely *originate* with this episode; it is more

likely that this episode served to *reinforce* preexisting perceptions. It is further possible that any feelings of hostility that Joseph
experienced from his siblings were in fact projections of his own
anger onto the siblings themselves. The plight of a crippled middle child would not have been a pleasant one in a crowded, penurious household where there was not enough to go around.

Despite the formidable difficulties in the retrospective appli-
cation of psychoanalytic understanding to an incomplete biographical record, the close scrutiny of a piece of original literature
such as *The Book of Mormon* may yet be a fruitful route to the in-
nermost thoughts and conflicts of its author. It is here, as Brodie
has discerned, that Joseph's struggles are played out in his realm
of fantasy and dictated in a kind of "free association." But just as
no analysis of a single dream can be complete, even when an experienced analyst is involved, any such examination of a piece of
literature will, of necessity, fall far short of full understanding and
may provoke honest debate.

There would seem to be room for disagreement with Brodie,
for instance, concerning the relative importance of fratricide and
patricide in the book. Although she is correct in identifying the
considerable importance of sibling rivalry, the affectionate relationships often expressed between fathers and sons in *The Book
of Mormon* should not be permitted to obscure the loathing toward father that accompanies such affection. The theme of patricide, the dark side of ambivalence toward the father, is indeed
very strong in *The Book of Mormon* but is often sufficiently disguised that it is not immediately recognizable.

A clear example of this ambivalence—father-love alongside
father-hatred—is the story of Laban, perhaps the best known and
best developed subplot of *The Book of Mormon,* and one expressed quite significantly at the book's very outset. In this short
vignette, Lehi and his family have fled into the wilderness and
have arrived at the seashore in their flight from Jerusalem, having
been warned in a vision that Jerusalem would be destroyed and
many of its inhabitants "should perish by the sword." Acting on
a second vision, Lehi directs his heroic young son Nephi to return
to Jerusalem with his brothers to obtain from the evil Laban the
engraved brass plates with the Judaic record and genealogy of the

family. Nephi's brother Laman first approaches Laban with the request but is angrily rebuffed and barely escapes with his life. The brothers then try to buy the plates with the wealth Lehi has left behind in the family's flight from Jerusalem, but Laban orders his servants to kill the brothers and take the money. The servants are successful in taking the brothers' money, but the brothers elude their pursuers by hiding in the "cavity of a rock." Nephi's evil brothers, Laman and Lemuel, beat Nephi with a rod until an angel scolds them for their actions. Nephi enters Jerusalem alone at night and finds Laban lying drunk on the ground. He admires Laban's wondrous sword with its hilt "of pure gold" and "exceedingly fine workmanship" and its blade "of the most precious steel." Nephi unsheaths Laban's sword from its scabbard. After much urging from "the Spirit" and after wrestling with his own conscience, Nephi lifts Laban's head by the hair and decapitates him. He dons Laban's clothes and sword and proceeds to Laban's home. There he encounters the treasurer Zoram, who sees the clothes and the sword, mistakes him for Laban, and unlocks the treasury, from which the two carry the brass plates out to Nephi's brothers. The brothers are initially terrified of Nephi, thinking he is Laban, but Nephi identifies himself to them and then skillfully persuades Zoram to join the family at the seashore. All return with the plates to Lehi and his wife.

Although this story is brimming with sibling rivalry, its main theme is patricide and can thus be best understood in a psychoanalytic context. What its author has done is a characteristic example of "splitting," a primitive defense mechanism commonly used by traumatized children. Joseph's ambivalence toward his father has been expressed in the literary device of dividing his father into two separate characters, both of whose names begin with the letter "L." (Indeed, Joseph, Jr. describes that the two are in fact related, both being descended from Joseph of the Old Testament.) In Lehi is seen all righteousness. Because of his goodness, God has chosen him alone to escape with his family, Noah-like, from impending destruction. God has special plans for Lehi and, perforce, his heroic son Nephi. Laban, on the other hand, is quintessentially evil. He is selfish, dishonest, greedy, rude, and cruel. He is also proud, wealthy, and in possession of a great treasure. Because of his remarkable sword, he is very powerful. Of course, anyone with so many vices and such a valuable treasure must be vulnerable to the wits of a clever lad, and Laban's intemperance ultimately leads to his ruin. And finally, were there any doubt that Laban is an evil-father personage, it is only necessary to recall the significance of his name. In the Book of Genesis, it will be recalled, the character Laban is the uncle who forces Jacob to work seven years to gain the hand of his beautiful daughter Rachel, only to give him instead the homely older sister Leah at the end of the time; this Laban requires seven more years of work before finally bequeathing Rachel's hand. A more deceitful and rivalrous paternal namesake would be hard to find.

Joseph, Jr. thus seems to have constructed a classic "overthrow" fantasy in this tale. It is a fair assumption that the climactic act of the story is a vivid reenactment of his final childhood operation, but with the roles reversed, as commonly occurs in boys' postoperative dreams.

The one-sided encounter with Laban, notably, takes place in the dark, perhaps a hidden message from the author's dissociated memories that the deed is not a noble one. (Could the darkness also represent the intensity of the patricidal fantasy as well?) The fact that the event occurs while Laban is sleeping spares the hero from having to look his adversary in the eye during the murder. Laban is portrayed as "fallen to earth," condemned by his own misdeeds. The only redeeming feature of the degraded Laban appears to be his awesome sword, described in superlative terms. Not only does Nephi confiscate the fearsome weapon from this surgeon/father representation but he destroys the representation with it as well. In performing the unthinkable act, the hero not only takes his revenge on his evil father but also carries the age-specific oedipal imagery into the fantasy. The act might be thought of as a double "castration." As decapitation is typically a representation of castration in male dream imagery, the confiscation of the sword and the decapitation with that very instrument thus seem to be dual representations of the unresolved oedipal anger symbolized by the surgery. This story is the most vivid reverse reenactment of Joseph's childhood operation in his writings. At this moment in the first chapter of the first book of *The Book of Mormon,* the central issues in Joseph Smith, Jr.'s conflict merge into a fused symbol; Dr. Nathan Smith's fearsome amputation knife takes on immense power as the mythical sword of Laban.

But it is the "splitting" of his father into two persons that permits Joseph Smith to allow the murder to occur in his story at all. As in the universal male child's fantasy, actually killing one's father is truly unthinkable. But if one can in some way protect the beloved father and kill only the loathsome part, the act is absolutely permissible. In fact, the good father, Lehi, will be enhanced by this action of his son the hero, Nephi, and the identification of the good son with his godlike father will in turn be increased.

Having disposed of Laban, Nephi puts on the dead man's clothes in an overt act of identification with the evil victim, most appropriate after the cold-blooded murder of an unconscious man. Nephi also states that he "did gird on [Laban's] armour about my loins." Having confiscated the terrible weapon in a turnabout of his own childhood nightmare, the author carries his fantasy to its logical extreme by transplanting the father's potent weapon to his young hero. The son is now sufficiently powerful to acquire the treasure because Laban's servant obeys when he "beheld the garments, and also the sword girted about my loins." The older brothers respond to the same ruse.

Thus does the sword of Laban—the terrifying specter of Nathan Smith's amputation knife, hiding just outside Joseph's conscious memory—become a key talisman in *The Book of Mormon,* for it will be seen again and again. The story of its capture surely sprang out of a dissociative trance. The sword subsequently appears in the book as a representation of invincible power, wielded by each hero in turn in the performance of triumphant acts. And as will be seen in Chapter 7, it will have a final purpose beyond *The Book of Mormon,* one that unites past and present in the fantasies of its creator.

This small anecdote concerning Laban is a revealing one in *The Book of Mormon* and the most literarily developed in an otherwise fairly tedious and shallow narrative. The fact that it occurs very early is highly significant for the degree of importance it represents in its author's world of fantasy. The episode provides a talisman for later use, and enormous power is bestowed on the character of the emerging hero.

There is yet another clue to the primacy of this story for its author, and that is its setting. This vignette does not occur in the promise of the New World; it occurs in the unresolved chaos of the Old. Nephi makes his perilous journey from the safe harbor of the seashore back to the site of the original chaos to perform the deed. It is as though he must assuage his anger by returning from the seashore to settle a score with his evil father before moving on. And this, of course, is precisely what Joseph Smith, Jr. must have fantasized during the dreadful days of seaside exile with his Uncle Jesse after the brutal trauma at the hands of his father and Dr. Nathan Smith. The disguise is thin.

Heroic Main Character

Despite the fact that *The Book of Mormon* traces a chronology over thousands of years, its author has nevertheless created a book with a single hero. As with the legendary phoenix, when one heroic central figure dies, another arises from the ashes to take his place. Sharing similar character structures, all have an air of invulnerability and resemble what Freud described as "His Majesty the Ego—the hero of all day-dreams and novels" (8). Nephi is Joseph as Holmes is Doyle as Hamlet is Shakespeare.

Nephi's personality has a dual nature, on the one hand powerful and on the other weak, humble, and childlike. The story of the encounter with Laban shows the hero's fearsome power. He is described as "large in stature," "an instrument in the hands of God," and "a ruler and a teacher over thy brethren." However, he is at the same time able to prophesy only because of his "plainness," is not "mighty in writing," but yet is able to write "notwithstanding my weakness."

To give greater definition to this duality, the author splits off the weak side into a younger brother whose name is, appropriately, Joseph. To this son the father Lehi says, "Thou wast born in the wilderness of mine afflictions; yea, in the days of my greatest sorrow, did thy mother bear thee." To the extent that Joseph Smith, Jr. was born just after his father's loss of the large dowry and the family farm and in the ignominy of land rental from his father-in-law, there is more than a little autobiographical truth to this. And in a likely reference to his childhood operation and the subsequent years on crutches, Joseph, Jr. has apparently fantasized of himself, "Out of weakness he shall be made strong." Joseph is further advised by Lehi, "Behold, thou are little; wherefore, hearken unto the words of thy brother Nephi," and the linkage between the two aspects of the hero's personality is thereby emphasized.

The introduction of a character named Joseph at this early stage in *The Book of Mormon* serves another valuable function for its author. It allows Joseph Smith, Jr. to link himself ancestrally through his father Joseph Smith, Sr., through this *The Book of Mormon* character Joseph, to Joseph of the Old Testament. In II Nephi 2, Lehi speaks of his own lineage back to Joseph of the Old Testament, and Lehi's son Joseph prophesies of the coming of Joseph Smith, Jr. ("And his name shall be called after me; and it shall be after the name of his father").

The link with Joseph of the Old Testament is hardly coincidental. The frequent references to this character as the author's ancestor throughout *The Book of Mormon* are strong evidence for a strong identification with him and his story. Joseph Smith, Jr. usually links himself with the Old Testament Joseph rather than to, in what would seem to be more logical links, the more prominent patriarchs Abraham or Isaac. The Joseph story, it will be recalled, is one of intense sibling rivalry. The fact that the Old Testament Joseph was the most beloved of his father's many sons is likely the wishful fantasy that Joseph Smith, Jr. carried of himself. Furthermore, the period of suffering in slavery that the ancient Joseph endured paralleled the period of prolonged lameness endured by Joseph, Jr. as a child. The ability to interpret the dreams of Pharaoh fits with his trauma-inspired self-image as a clairvoyant. And finally, the triumphant domination that the Old Testament Joseph exercised over the fate of his father and brothers after their humble pleas for food during the famine was again for Joseph, Jr. a ready identification with his wishful fantasies.

Included among these many anecdotes of invincibility are the subsequent heroic characters Alma and Amulek, who, while "bound with cords" in prison, break their shackles as the prison falls down, with all their enemies being killed but they themselves spared. In another story a mob assaults heroic Samuel with stones and arrows at point-blank range and yet fails to strike him with even a single missile.

Joseph Smith, Jr. chooses to make reprise the original auto-biographical name Nephi for the dominant heroic character immediately preceding this climactic moment of Jesus Christ's arrival in the New World. The event is surrounded by cataclysms of nature and a miraculous bodily descent of Jesus from the sky. *The Book of Mormon* Jesus, however, has a personality that is not qualitatively distinguishable from that of the serial hero throughout the rest of the book; the difference is merely one of degree.

Central to this personality is Jesus' relationship to God his Father. Although the New Testament Jesus on occasion speaks paternally of God (and then often in the plural possessive [e.g., "Our Father in heaven"]), *The Book of Mormon* Jesus often demonstrates the sort of subservient, powerless, and passive role vis-à-vis his Father that the other *The Book of Mormon* heroes—and indeed Joseph Smith, Jr. himself—typically show. In fact, much of the time, *The Book of Mormon* Jesus seems even to excuse himself from responsibility for some of his Father's actions and suggests, in effect, that the listeners would have to ask his Father themselves. In dealing with the puzzling circumstance that he failed to disclose during his former life in Galilee that he would soon descend from the sky in a public spectacle 10,000 miles away, *The Book of Mormon* Jesus blithely absolves himself from the need for such explanation by blaming his father:

> And not at any time hath the Father given me commandment
> that I should tell it unto your brethren at Jerusalem; . . .
> I was commanded to say no more of the Father concerning
> this thing unto them. (III Nephi 7, p. 486)

But even though his Father forms a convenient foil from time to time, there is no question who holds the power to manipulate both his Father and his Father's followers:

> And the Holy Ghost beareth record of the Father and me; and the Father giveth the Holy Ghost unto the children of men, *because of me.* (III Nephi 13, p. 510)

> Therefore if ye call upon the Father, for the church, if it be in my name, the Father will hear you. (III Nephi 12, p. 507)

The melding of traditional Christian theology and paternal rivalry in *The Book of Mormon* Jesus is subtle but unmistakable in many such passages.

Jesus' appearance in the New World in *The Book of Mormon* carries far greater significance, however, because it reveals how Joseph Smith, Jr. associated himself uniquely with the suffering figure of Jesus of the cross. In view of the impact of the religious revivals of his adolescent years superimposed on the emotional trauma of his childhood surgery, it would have been unlikely that just such a sense of identification would not have developed on some level of consciousness. Indeed, there is some historical testimony supporting this association. Eber D. Howe quotes a Smith neighbor, Hezekiah M'Kune, as stating that "in conversation with Joseph Smith Jr., he (Smith) said he was nearly equal to Jesus Christ . . ." (9). A second neighbor, Levi Lewis, "testifies that he heard Smith say he (Smith) was as good as Jesus Christ;—that it was as bad to injure him as it was to injure Jesus Christ" (10). (Note the reference to injury.) Again, there is continuing evidence that Joseph's childhood operation played an important role in this identification. In III Nephi 12 (p. 508), Joseph Smith has Jesus state: ". . . therefore none entereth into his rest, save it be those who have washed their garments in my blood, because of their faith, and the repentance of all their sins, and their faithfulness unto the end."

In Chapter 3 it was pointed out that children's immobilization after surgery is strongly connected with a sense of "atonement for some naughtiness or sin, a price they had to pay for the premium of later health" (11). By suffering through the treatment, the child feels he or she has atoned for his or her naughtiness and is thereby restored. But immobilization is merely a passive form of "punishment"; Joseph was not so lucky. He had experienced three times in close succession the simultaneous horrors of fiery pain and the specter of his own blood gushing over his bed, his attackers, and himself.

In this context it is small wonder that the metaphor of washing garments in Christ's blood appears repeatedly throughout Joseph's writings and speeches. He knew about restraint with arms outstretched, about nails driven into extremities, about the thrust of a sword into one's body, and about the shedding of one's blood in betrayal by one's own people. He knew about guilt and atonement. At some level of his psyche he knew all too well about the crucifixion, and in his narcissistic perception of himself he found it but a small step to establish identification with Jesus Christ. In *The Book of Mormon,* in psychoanalytic terms, Nephi and Jesus are both Joseph Smith, Jr.

Father-Identification

One of the strongest themes running throughout *The Book of Mormon* is that of father-identification, the tightly bonded affiliation a son feels toward his father in thought, status, and fate. This theme of father-identification was of sufficient importance to Joseph Smith, Jr. that he chose to open *The Book of Mormon* with it: "I, Nephi, having been born of goodly parents, therefore I was taught somewhat in all the learning of my father . . . yea, I make a record in the language of my father . . ." (I Nephi 1, p. 5). One gains the impression that the serial hero feels a sense of legitimacy throughout *The Book of Mormon* by identifying with his father. It is as though the childlike hero needs reassurance of his own worth through identification with his noble father.

This theme provides the basis for the strong patriarchal organization of society in *The Book of Mormon,* wherein power and authority are virtually always passed from father to son, or at least passed in paternal fashion from a senior to a junior male. It also gives rise to a patriarchal pattern of proper names that reinforces this identification. It is usual, for example, that the particular son who happens to possess the father's name will eventually be the one to inherit the mantle of leadership regardless of birth order (as with Joseph, Jr. himself). On occasion, as with the heroic character Mormon, although the reader never encounters the father at all, the author seems to be compelled to imbue the hero with father-identification:

> And I, Mormon, being a descendent of Nephi, (and my father's name was Mormon,) . . . (Mormon 1, p. 519)

> Condemn me not because of mine imperfections; neither my father because of his imperfection . . . (Mormon 4, p. 538)

But along with this sense of legitimacy accorded to the son by virtue of his affiliation with his father is a subtle message that the son is somehow the greater of the two. Nephi writes on the plates an account of his own life but only an abridgment of the record of his father. The most revered Lehi had to be "truly chastened because of his murmuring against the Lord," whereas his son Nephi had never doubted the Lord. And it is not likely that Joseph Smith's mere unfamiliarity with proper grammar produced Nephi's phrase "I and my father." Sons always seem to outdo their fathers in *The Book of Mormon.*

Perhaps the ultimate example of father-identification is seen in the apparition of Jesus Christ speaking to the brother of Jared:

> Behold, I am Jesus Christ. *I am the Father and the Son* . . .
> . . . he that will not believe me will not believe the Father who sent me. For, behold, *I am the Father,* I am the light, and the life, and the truth of the world. (Ether 1, pp. 544, 547) (emphasis added)

This final passage stands the traditional view of the Trinity on its head and negates the clear and necessary distinction between God the Father and Jesus Christ during the latter's visit to the Americas described in *The Book of Mormon.* Jesus' claim to be his own father in this instance seems a manifestation of both the father-identification and the unresolved father jealousy of the book's author. Being Jesus Christ may be the greatest attainment of a man, but it still holds that accursed subservient position to one's Father. In the Book of Ether in *The Book of Mormon*, Joseph Smith, Jr. overcomes even that limitation.[4]

Evil Father and Patricide

The opposite face of father imagery in *The Book of Mormon* is that of intense loathing—not arising from but certainly reinforced through the author's surgery. The prototypical patricidal event in Nephi's murder of Laban in the first chapter of the first book is a case in point. There are many more such examples in *The Book of Mormon*, though it is often necessary to peel back the subliminal disguises of kings, jailers, and clergy to see the father lurking within.

It is noteworthy, for instance, that the first person to die among the righteous party leaving Jerusalem in the opening chapters of *The Book of Mormon* is Nephi's father-in-law Ishmael. It is interesting both because he is a close father-substitute whom the author gets out of the way early and because Isaac Hale, the threatening, real-life counterpart of Ishmael, shares the first two letters of his name (the first three if one counts the initial of his surname). Immediately following the death of Ishmael from natural causes, Nephi's brothers and brothers-in-law are described as plotting to murder both Nephi and his father. Did the placement of this subplot to murder Nephi immediately after Ishmael's death represent an expression of the guilt felt by the author over his fantasy of wish-fulfillment toward Isaac Hale? Judging from what is recorded of the relationship between the two, it hardly seems surprising that Joseph arranges the father-in-law's demise at the first available moment.

---

[4] It is noteworthy that this view of a fused Father-Son deity was put forward by Joseph Smith, Jr. an additional time during a May 1831 prophecy to a group of church elders: ". . . you are of them that my Father hath given me; and none of them that my Father hath given me shall be lost; and the Father and I are one; I am in the Father and the Father in me . . ." (12) (emphasis added).

This guilt surrounding a patricidal act, seen both here and in the murder of Laban, can always be found lurking in the drama surrounding every such event in *The Book of Mormon* in one form or another. Often it takes the form of some last-minute reprieve for the doomed father or father-representative. An example of such a reprieve is seen in Alma 12 within the disguised imagery of Joseph's childhood trauma. In this scene the newly converted Lamanite king, Lamoni, is traveling with the righteous young Nephite hero Ammon when they encounter Lamoni's father, the most evil "king over all the land." When Lamoni refuses his father's order to kill Ammon, his father draws his sword to kill his own son for disobedience. Ammon stands forward to condemn the evil father: "Behold, thou shalt not slay thy son. . . . for if thou shouldst slay thy son, (he being an innocent man,) his blood would cry from the ground" (Alma 12, p. 281).

The evil father-king then "stretched forth his hand" to kill Ammon only to find that Ammon "smote his arm that he could not use it" (Alma 12, p. 281) in another wish-fulfilling reenactment of the childhood trauma. This oedipal act of functional dismemberment of an erected extremity is followed by the king's agreeing to a plea-bargain to save his life. In *The Book of Mormon,* symbolic dismemberment of the father is acceptable as turnabout vengeance for the author's own most dreadful experience; murder, however, is too much.

In Alma 21, there is yet another variant of the same patricidal fantasy. The treacherous Amalickiah is able to get rid of the reigning Lamanite king. Significantly, he does not kill the king himself; instead one of his nameless servants stabs the king in the heart. Amalickiah then encounters the queen, seeks her favor, and marries her. (Two chapters later Amalickiah will receive a javelin in the heart while sleeping.)

One suspects that some external event in Joseph Smith's life provoked an unusual eruption of patricidal anger during his composition of the third and fourth chapters of the Book of Ether, for the tales told in these nine pages possess waves of such fury. The convoluted story contains eight vignettes of sons overthrowing fathers, three narrow "escapes" from patricide, two patricides by surrogate sons (not actual sons), two planned beheadings, and the starvation of a son in prison.[5]

In the exception that is to prove the rule, these incidents are followed by the only literal face-to-face patricide in *The Book of Mormon*. Heth actually murders his father, Com, with Com's own sword to usurp the kingdom. But this act brings about a plague of "poisonous serpents," which not only kill many people but chase all the livestock out of the country. Heth and many others die in the resulting famine. This "revenge of the serpents," with its oedipal overtones, seems likely to be an expression of the author's guilt over the event of patricide.

The final such fantasy in the climactic chaos leading to the ultimate annihilation is described in a writing of Mormon to his son in which "the husbands and fathers of those women and children they have slain" are described as feeding "the women upon the flesh of their husbands, and the children upon the flesh of their fathers . . ." (Moroni 9, p. 584).

Joseph's fantasies, played out in his writings, reveal a great deal about the objects of his repressed anger. It is the father who is the most loathed; brothers do slightly better.

Joseph Smith's Childhood Operation

Those themes in *The Book of Mormon* discussed thus far—the nature of the heroic main character, the powerful ambivalence toward the author's father, and sibling rivalry—reflect major issues troubling Joseph Smith, Jr. But since these are universal themes in literary and artistic expression, it should not be surprising to discover them, nor should it be surprising to find that they have

---

[5] As Bettelheim points out in his discussion of Hansel and Gretel, "A small child, awakening hungry in the darkness of the night, feels threatened by complete rejection and desertion, which he experiences in the form of fear of starvation. By projecting their inner anxiety onto those they fear might cut them off, Hansel and Gretel are convinced that their parents plan to starve them to death" (13). In reading of this starvation episode, one can only wonder about the deprivation experienced by Joseph Smith, Jr. during the poverty-stricken years of his childhood.

struck harmonious chords with millions of *The Book of Mormon* readers. All humans struggle with these issues to some degree, and Joseph's literary disguises are sufficiently translucent that many readers evidently sense concord with the author's struggle. The communication succeeds.

But if, as suggested in previous chapters, many of these and other issues seen in *The Book of Mormon* have risen to primacy as a result of Joseph's childhood trauma, it would be expected that the text of the book would reflect not only a disproportionate emphasis on these themes but also some more direct allusions to the actual incident of trauma itself. This, it turns out, is abundantly the case.

An example is the state of mind represented in the following speech by the heroic Jacob:

> I can tell you concerning your thoughts, how that ye are beginning to labor in sin. . . .
>
> Wherefore, it burdeneth my soul, that I should be constrained . . . to admonish you, according to your crimes, *to enlarge the wounds of those which are already wounded, instead of consoling and healing their wounds*; and those which have not been wounded, instead of feasting upon the pleasing word of God, have *daggers placed to pierce their souls, and wound their delicate minds*. But, notwithstanding the greatness of the task, I must do according to the strict commands of God, and tell you concerning your wickedness and abominations, in the presence of the pure in heart, and the broken heart, and *under the glance of the piercing eye of the Almighty God*. (Jacob 2, p. 125) (emphasis added)

The physical imagery alone unmistakably refers to Joseph's brutal operations. Here, as elsewhere, his reenactment is expressed through a theological disguise.

It appears from the first italicized portion of the passage that Joseph remained yet hostile and ignorant of the necessity of Dr. Nathan Smith's debriding his leg wound. He laments the fact that Dr. Smith's treatment enlarged the wound "instead of consoling and healing," suggesting that he felt himself to be the victim of an unjustified assault on these occasions and had no comprehension of the therapeutic value of his operative treatment. This passage appears to contradict those claims of his mother that Joseph had asked the doctors to proceed at her therapeutic suggestion.

And finally, the imagery itself is noteworthy. The daggers pierce "souls" and "minds" as much as "wounds"— and all under the "glance of the piercing eye of the Almighty God." This final metaphor combines the physical nature of the "piercing" scalpel, the probing eye that must have discerned young Joseph's age-appropriate fantasies, with the reference to the all-powerful father/surgeon who watched and condoned the operation, held Joseph fast against his struggling, and presumably arranged the punishment in the first place. The physical pain and humiliation of Joseph's brutal operations reemerge from dissociated memory as a religious theme in this passage and throughout his writing. The disguise is effective, the imagery is powerful, and the impact is historical.

A further metaphor with all the same nuances of meaning is found in one of Joseph's prophecies delivered in 1830 in Fayette, New York:

> Open ye your ears and hearken to the voice of the Lord your God, whose word is quick and powerful, sharper than a two-edged sword, to the dividing asunder of the joints and marrow, soul and spirit; and is a discerner of the thoughts and intents of the heart. (14)

Again, the physical description of Joseph's operation is unmistakable, especially in the reference to bone marrow, and the broader significance for the operation as a discovery and punishment of evil acts is equally clear. The haunting centrality of the sword is again evident.

An additional reference to the surgery-as-redemption theme is graphically spelled out in another 1830 prophecy given by Joseph in Manchester, New York. One can almost visualize the white-as-if-transparent prophet spewing the words out of his dissociated memory:

> I command you to repent—repent *lest I smite you by the rod of my mouth, and by my wrath, and by my anger, and*

your sufferings be sore—how sore you know not! how ex-
quisite you know not! yea, how hard to bear you know not!
For, behold, I, God, have suffered these things for all, that
they might not suffer, if they would repent; but if they
would not repent, they must suffer even as I; which suffer-
ing caused myself, even God, the greatest of all, to tremble
because of pain, and to bleed at every pore, and to suffer
both body and spirit, and would that I might not drink the
bitter cup . . . [Did young Joseph accept the proffered
brandy from Nathan Smith after all, or did he perhaps reject
it because it tasted badly?]

   . . . confess your sins, lest you suffer these punishments
which I have spoken . . .

   . . . for they cannot bear meat now, but milk they must receive; . . . [Could this be an allusion to Nathan Smith's postoperative dietary instructions to Lucy?] (15) (emphasis
added)

And what would be the mark left by those abominable
thoughts, the terrifying symbol of the aftermath, forever stained
into the canvas of Joseph's psyche?

> And now I ask of you, my brethren, how will any of you feel,
> if ye shall stand before the bar of God, having your garments
> stained with blood, and all manner of filthiness? . . . that ye
> are guilty of all manner of wickedness? (Alma 3, p. 234)

The metaphor of blood-stained garments as a symbol representing sin echoes with some monotony throughout *The Book of
Mormon* and through Joseph's later prophecies as recorded in
the *Doctrine and Covenants.* The need for "spotless garments" is
often described in frenetic terms. To make garments spotless, as
the metaphor continues, "your garments have been cleansed and
made white, through the blood of Christ, which will come to re-
deem his people from their sins" (Alma 3, pp. 234–235).

   Again, the notion of atonement for naughtiness appears, as it
did in the studies of immobilized children described in Chapter 3.
But for Joseph, this initial vague perception of suffering-as-
atonement has become elaborated into a grand superstructure of

fantasy wherein his own blood and that of Jesus Christ have become somehow commingled. Later, as the *The Book of Mormon*
Jesus prophesies of the coming of Joseph Smith, direct reference
is made to Joseph's surgery:

> But, behold, the life of my servant [Joseph Smith] shall be in
> my hand; therefore they shall not hurt him, although he
> shall be marred because of them. Yet I will heal him, for I will
> shew unto them that my wisdom is greater than the cunning
> of the Devil. (III Nephi 9, p. 500)

Finally, to complete the remaining link through the opera-
tions to Joseph's identification with Jesus Christ, a jump beyond
The Book of Mormon may be made to a prophecy by Joseph
Smith, given shortly thereafter in 1831: "I am Christ, and in mine
own name, by virtue of the blood which I have spilt, have
I pleaded before the Father for them" (16).

Having completed the linkage of himself to Jesus Christ, Joseph
may now repeatedly play out the biblical metaphor of purification
by his own "blood of Christ." The metaphor is usually presented in
his writings in a curious twist of the Lady Macbeth format. The
bloodstain (originally guilt over his own fantasies about his operations, but later elaborated to symbolize all sin) needs to be meticu-
lously eradicated from the garments as a sign that the atonement
through suffering has triumphed. But paradoxically, the sin can be
removed only by cleansing in the blood of Christ. Joseph, in a pattern characteristic of childhood trauma, seems to have taken the
horrifying childhood specter of being covered in his own blood
and *split it into two opposing parts*—one good and one evil—not
unlike his splitting of Lehi and Laban. The evil blood is that on his
own garments shed at the time of the awful surgical trauma,
brought about by all of his own forbidden thoughts. The good
blood is that symbolizing the atonement achieved by this suffering
and linked through identification with Jesus Christ as a natural extension of himself. With this construct firmly embedded in his
mind, there could be little doubt that he himself was central to the
redemption of mankind—or at least of that part of it who would acknowledge his omnipotence.

On a less theological note, *The Book of Mormon* provides further evidence to suggest that Lucy Smith's account of Joseph's final operation was incomplete. During the opening journey over the ocean to the Americas, for instance, Nephi describes how he was treated:

> Laman and Lemuel did take me and bind me with cords, and they did treat me with much harshness . . . that I could not move, my brethren began to see that the judgment of God was upon them . . .
> . . . wherefore, they came unto me and loosed the bands which was upon my wrists, and behold, they had much swollen, exceedingly; and also, my ancles were much swollen, and great was the soreness thereof. (I Nephi 5, pp. 48–49)

It is noteworthy that the binding with cords is specifically limited to the wrists and ankles, although it was done "insomuch that I could not move." It does not require much imagination to conclude that the only position in which both of these conditions holds is that of being spread-eagled, as though attached to the four corners of a bedframe. This is almost certainly the position Dr. Nathan Smith and his medical students would have been accustomed to using as the first step in immobilizing a struggling child on whose leg they wished to operate. As to the clear physical description of the aftereffects of pain and swelling in the wrists and ankles, it is further testimony that Joseph "had been there."

The metaphors of physical bondage abound throughout *The Book of Mormon* and through Joseph's subsequent prophecies. Although the most common phrase is "bound with cords," almost certainly the means used by Dr. Nathan Smith, there is occasional embellishment of the metaphor to chains (as was the case in a quotation earlier in this section), and even to handcuffs, shackles, and "the fetters of hell."

Further probable descriptions of Joseph's leg wounds are to be found in a prophecy delivered by a white-countenanced prophet in August 1830 in Harmony, Pennsylvania:

Wherefore, I, the Lord God, will send forth flies upon the
face of the earth, which shall take hold of the inhabitants
thereof, and shall eat their flesh, and shall cause maggots to
come in upon them, and their tongues shall be stayed that
they shall not utter against me, and their flesh shall fall from
off their bones. (17)

Even modern surgeons periodically observe maggots in open
sores of longstanding duration such as burns and leg ulcers. This
author has seen them on several occasions in less-than-optimal
hygienic conditions. In truth, maggots are enormously beneficial
for wound care because they are very effective in removing dead
tissue. In any case, the prevailing hygienic conditions in rural New
England before 1820 would have virtually guaranteed that maggots would have visited Joseph's chronic leg wound, and it is no
doubt useful that they did so. The dead flesh would indeed have
fallen off his tibia to permit the slow healing process to com-
mence.

For an additional bit of speculation about a theme in *The
Book of Mormon* related to Joseph's operation, attention is directed to the anti-Masonic movement reviewed on pp. 89–90. Although at first glance this theme appears to be a self-evident,
self-explanatory, and self-contained motif, there may be more to
it than Joseph's simple parroting of the prevailing community
sentiment about an unpopular group. Although the actual evidence for this hypothesis is thin, it is possible that the idea of evil
"secret combinations," Joseph's code word for the Masonic order, may have had an antecedent in Joseph's early life. Is it possible that Joseph regarded the surgeon and his retinue of medical
students in such fashion? Were they conspiring to continue their
periodic satanic visits of cruelty to his bedroom? What did Joseph in his sleep-deprived state make of their group dynamics,
and how did he think the doctors were organized? If Joseph at
the age of seven did regard the doctors as being involved in some
form of secret conspiracy, then the rumors about the Masons in
his young adult life would have fallen on fertile soil. This might
explain why this single contemporary political issue was singled
out for such emphasis:

> [T]he Lord worketh not in secret combinations, neither does he will that man should shed blood, but in all things hath forbidden it, from the beginning of man . . .
>
> . . . yea, even the sword of the justice of the eternal God, shall fall upon you, to your overthrow and destruction . . .
>
> . . . ye shall awake to a sense of your awful situation, because of this secret combination which shall be among you, or wo be to it, because of the blood of them which have been slain: for they cry from the dust for vengeance upon it, and also upon those who build it up. (Ether 3, p. 554)

Is this a reference to persecution by a small conspiracy of cruel blood-shedding surgeons or merely an allusion to Masonry? The case is suggestive.

The final theme that shows a clear but convoluted linkage to Joseph's operation is a pair of references in *The Book of Mormon* to the issue of children and their relation to sin. The first of these references occurs during the valedictory speech of King Benjamin delivered from a tower just after he has transferred power to his son Mosiah and given him the plates of brass and the sword of Laban:

> [T]he law of Moses availeth nothing, except it were through the atonement of [Christ's] blood; and even if it were possible that little children could sin, they could not be saved . . . the blood of Christ atoneth for their sins . . . the infant perisheth not, that dieth in his infancy; but men drinketh damnation to their own souls, except they humble themselves, and become as little children . . . in and through the atoning blood of Christ, . . . and becometh as a child, submissive, meek, humble, patient, full of love, willing to submit to all things which the Lord seeth fit to inflict upon him, *even as a child doth submit to his father.* (Mosiah 1, p. 161) (emphasis added)

In this verbose passage Joseph speaks of the innocence of children alongside the issue of blood atonement. The final words of the passage refer to the passivity of childhood, especially with reference to his father. The linkage lies less in the actual text than in the fact that the subjects are juxtaposed through their proximity to each other.

The second reference to childhood sin is in a letter from Mormon to his son Moroni in which there is contained a lengthy condemnation of infant baptism. The passage opens with Christ speaking:

> Behold, I came into the world not to call the righteous, but sinners to repentance; the whole need no physician, but they that are sick; wherefore little children are whole, for they are not capable of committing sin; wherefore the curse of Adam is taken from them in me, that it hath no power over them: and the law of circumcision is done away in me. (Moroni 8, p. 581)

In this passage childhood sin is addressed in the same sentence as physicians and circumcision, the common themes of Joseph's childhood trauma. Although few clues are provided other than the literary juxtaposition of the concepts in the two passages, the assumption may be made that the issue of sin in children was related in Joseph's mind in some way to blood atonement and to submissiveness of children to their fathers, to physicians, and to circumcision.

In addition to its ritual significance, circumcision is, of course, a symbolic expression of an assault on the penis by the father—a "castration" event endured by a submissive child. More specifically, in the Judaic tradition it signifies "the omnipotent and threatening character of the God who demanded it" (18), thus reinforcing the significance of the rite as an act of submission to powerful father figures. The circumcision compact, enforced by symbolic castration, promises privilege and protection in return for obedience. But since, as Bettelheim states, "only where the punitive figure of an adult looms large will the child easily make the mental transition from circumcision to castration anxiety" (19), it is not surprising that Joseph writes in the above passage of his fantasy of abolishing the rite of circumcision. He suggests that adults need to protect children from circumcision, with all of its fearsome connotations, by denying to children their very capacity for sin. The fantasy seems to be another expression of wish-fulfillment related to his own childhood nightmare.

The Scalpel

Nathan Smith's terrifying amputation knife seems always to have been Joseph's central visual symbol for his operations. The sword's fiery plunge into his tissues on three separate occasions (four if one includes the abscess in his armpit) assured its primacy. Imagery in *The Book of Mormon* that represents the weapon itself needs to be recognized, especially since that imagery appears to carry the hidden oedipal symbolism of Laban's sword. Although Brodie and other biographers have long noted the theme of phallicism in Joseph's creative work, it is tempting to overinterpret these symbols, especially when remembering Freud's broad definition of phallic disguises as "all elongated objects, sticks, tree-trunks, and umbrellas (on account of the stretching up which might be compared to an erection), all elongated and sharp weapons, knives, daggers, and pikes" (20). Keeping in mind Freud's own famous caveat that some of these cigars may be only cigars, it is nonetheless important to suggest a few interpretations.

The oft-repeated adjective "stiffnecked" does indeed mean stubborn, but it is evidently far more appealing to Joseph than any less graphic substitutes, if one views the frequency of its use in *The Book of Mormon* and the later prophecies. When God assists or protects men in their tasks in Joseph's writings, he "makes bare his arm" (Did Nathan Smith roll up his sleeve before picking up the scalpel in Joseph's dissociated memory?), "makes flesh his arm," places "his arm over all the earth," "lengthens out his arm," or "extends his arm of mercy to men, protecting them against the fiery darts of the adversary." On the other hand, when God behaves as a vengeful evil father, his "sword of justice hangs over" evildoers and often falls on them if they do not repent. The fused imagery of phallicism and the amputation knife is seen in these oft-repeated metaphors.

At times, sensuality appears to accompany the violent aspects of the imagery. Among several possible sexualized metaphors found in Joseph's writings is the following passage from an 1831 prophecy:

> Then shall the arm of the Lord fall upon the nations, and
> then shall the Lord set his foot upon this mount, and it shall
> cleave in twain, and the earth shall tremble and reel to and
> fro. (21)

The metaphor is even more suggestive when a phrase from the
The Book of Mormon is elaborated into a later prophecy:

> Yea, verily, verily I say unto you, that the field is white already
> to harvest; wherefore, thrust in your sickles, and reap with
> all your might, mind, and strength. (22)

On the other hand, the same images are often used as weapons
in the performance of violent and threatening acts of God in a manner that similarly recalls the nature of Joseph's encounter with Dr.
Nathan Smith. Such is the case when Nephi says of the Gentiles,
"[T]hey shall war among themselves, and the sword of their own
hands shall fall upon their own heads, and they shall be drunken
with their own blood" (I Nephi 7, p. 57). Or, as Nephi's brother Jacob says of God, "O that he would shew you that he can pierce you,
and with one glance of his eye, he can smite you to the dust" (Jacob
2, p. 8). And when the Spirit is withdrawn from a sinner, the poor
deserted man "is left unto himself, to kick against the pricks; to per-
secute the saints, and to fight against God" (23). When Joseph
Smith's follower William Law is told by Joseph in a later prophecy
that "he shall be led in paths where the poisonous serpent cannot
lay hold upon his heel" (24), the anatomic proximity to Joseph's
own childhood assault is perhaps more than coincidental. The
phrases "prick their hearts" and "hearts . . . pierced with deep
wounds" appear to have a similar connotation.

There is a further significance of phallic symbolism in Joseph's
writings as well—that of a representation of power. This aspect of
the meaning of such symbolism is liberally dispersed throughout
The Book of Mormon, especially in view of events that occur at the
tops of towers. King Benjamin and Helaman's son Nephi both address the multitudes from atop towers. King Limhi discovers the
invading Lamanite armies from his vantage point on top of a
tower, enabling him to organize a successful preemptive attack.
The "wicked and perverse" Zoramites worship from the top of the

Holy Stand, "a place built up in the centre of their synagogue, a place of standing, which was high above the head; and the top thereof would only admit one person" (Alma 16, p. 311). (The name of this tower is Rameumptom, close enough to "ram-upped-em" to bear passing mention.) In each of these instances, a rodlike symbol is used in some fashion to represent power on be-half of the person associated with it.

The *rod* is a particularly important symbol in *The Book of Mormon*. It is a representation of power that carries with it all the con-notations known to Joseph Smith, Sr., to Joseph Smith, Jr., and to the transcriptionist Oliver Cowdery from the days of the forked stick and the treasure hunts. The phallic symbolism of the divin-ing rod is obvious, of course, since its motion is activated upon discovery of its "treasure." Although the rod is occasionally seen as a weapon, as when Laman and Lemuel smite Nephi with a rod, or in the passage, "he shall smite the earth with the rod of his mouth" (II Nephi 12, p. 117), it is more usually seen as a symbol of power and privilege, as with a king's scepter. The rod of iron ap-pearing in Lehi's dream was interpreted by Nephi as representing "the word of God. . . . [N]either could the temptations and the fiery darts of the adversary, overpower them unto blindness, to lead them away to destruction" (I Nephi 4, p. 37). There is even a confrontation between such symbols in this particular passage, with the rod of iron triumphing over the "fiery darts."

Joseph Smith, Jr. also associates himself directly with the rod by providing a pointed prophecy of his own coming in *The Book of Mormon*. Nephi's brother Joseph proclaims of the future author, "[T]he Lord hath said, I will raise up a Moses; and I will give power unto him in a rod; and I will give judgment unto him in writing." It may be assumed that Joseph Smith, Jr. felt that he was "chosen" both because he identified with his father in assuming the gift of the divining rod and because such a sense of clairvoy-ance is a frequent delusion of the posttraumatic mindset. This association was a natural one for Joseph in his powerful identifi-cation with his father. The metaphor fits naturally into the context of father-identification.

Nor can the sword of Laban be overlooked. From its original capture at Joseph's supreme moment of dissociative fantasy, it serves as protector of the righteous and as the principal talisman of power in *The Book of Mormon*. Nephi in fact, "did take the sword of Laban, and after the manner of it did make many swords, lest by any means the people which were now called Lamanites, should come upon us and destroy us" (II Nephi 4, p. 72). The sword is passed along with the records engraved on the plates from leader to leader in patriarchal fashion. Periodically, Joseph provides reminders that the power continues, as when "king Benjamin gathered together his armies, and he did stand against them; and he did fight with the strength of his own arm, with the sword of Laban" (Words of Mormon 1, p. 152). After being passed from King Benjamin to his son Mosiah, the sword is no longer mentioned directly in *The Book of Mormon* but will later play an important role for its author.

One final symbol for the amputation knife in *The Book of Mormon* is worth mentioning at this stage, for it will be mentioned later, in Chapter 8, in the context of discussion of temple rites. Joseph takes particular note of the "flaming sword" left with cherubim by God at the east end of the Garden of Eden to keep Adam from the tree of life. Although the sword is usually regarded as a relatively insignificant feature of the story of Adam, Joseph promotes it to center stage. The metaphor seems more meaningful to him because of personal experience.

Anxiety About Dismemberment

The mere appearance of knifelike symbols in the story is, of course, insufficient to support a thesis that a horrible trauma in childhood was a driving force in the personality that created *The Book of Mormon*. The special focus of dismemberment imagery must also be abundant for the case to be supported, and Joseph does not disappoint. But again, each symbol for dismemberment must be recognized in its panoply of disguises. The story of Laban has already been described as a vivid patricidal/castration fantasy, as has the encounter of Ammon with Lamoni's evil father-king.

Another example is seen in the manner in which Lamoni

comes to be impressed with Ammon in the first place. Ammon is an enslaved Nephite tending sheep for King Lamoni. When a band of ruffians scatters the king's flocks at their watering place, Ammon takes the ruffians on single-handedly. After killing a few of them with well-thrown stones, Ammon is subjected to a curious attack:

> . . . seeing that they could not hit him with their stones, they came forth with clubs to slay him. But behold, every man that lifted his club to smite Ammon, he smote off their arms with his sword; for he did withstand their blows by smiting their arms with the edge of his sword, insomuch that they began to be astonished. . . . Now six of them had fallen by the sling, but he slew none save it were their leader; and he smote off as many of their arms as was lifted against him, and they were not a few . . . and then went in unto the king, bearing the arms which had been smote off by the sword of Ammon . . . for a testimony of the things which they had done. (Alma 12, pp. 272–273)

This passage is sufficiently transparent that it needs little embellishment in view of what is known of young boys' postsurgical fantasies. Each threatening arm with a club is severed by an even mightier sword wielded by the hero. And what greater manner of introduction to a king-father could be fantasized than to show him a bag of limbs that had been amputated by his young subject? Any king-father gazing on these would indeed see the wisdom in submitting to such an invincible lad. The fantasy is a wish-fulfilling reenactment of the childhood operations but with the roles reversed.

The description of a particularly bloody battle between the Nephites and Lamanites seems to express anxiety over dismemberment in yet another way. The Nephites are described as undergoing elaborate construction of protective armor, in contrast to the Lamanites, who are covered only with loinskins. The outcome of the battle is described as follows:

> . . . but it was more dreadful on the part of the Lamanites; for their nakedness was exposed to the heavy blows of the

Nephites, with their swords and their cimeters, which brought death almost at every stroke: while on the other hand, there was now and then a man fell among the Nephites, by their swords, and the loss of blood; they being shielded from the more vital parts of the body, or the more vital parts of the body being shielded from the strokes of the Lamanites, by their breast-plates, and their arm-shields, and their head-plates. (Alma 20, p. 343)

In addition to the fear of damaging "vital parts" expressed in this passage is something perhaps even more interest. Did Joseph, who was not writing by his own hand, inadvertently let a Freudian slip creep into his dictation? He specifically uses the phrase "they being shielded *from* the more vital parts of the body," but perhaps indicating by the subsequent use of the word "or" that he had recognized his misstatement and substituted the clause that follows, in which "the more vital parts of the body being shielded from the strokes of the Lamanites." Did Joseph in the first clause unwittingly reveal his less-than-conscious perception of the phallus as weapon? The fact that the phrasing slipped out at the moment when he was ruminating over a threat to "vital parts" is a credible symbolic replication of his dissociated fantasies. "Children who have been overstimulated," Shengold points out, "tend to see the adult penis as an organ that can effectively discharge cannibalistic overexcitation and can bite" (25).

In this frame of mind, Joseph dictated a counterattack by the Lamanites, who

yea, . . . did fight like dragons; and many of the Nephites were slain by their hands; yea, for they did smite in two many of their head-plates; and they did pierce many of their breast-plates; and they did smite off many of their arms; and thus the Lamanites did smite in their fierce anger. (Alma 20, p. 344)

These dismemberment-filled passages suggest origin within a dissociative trance of their author.

The climactic event of the battle follows a few verses later in a dramatic confrontation between the two leaders:

[Zerahemnah] was angry with Moroni, and he rushed forward that he might slay Moroni; but as he raised his sword,
behold, one of Moroni's soldiers smote it even to the earth;
and it broke by the hilt; and he also smote Zerahemnah, that
he took off his scalp, and it fell to the earth. . . .

And it came to pass that the soldier which stood by, which
smote off the scalp of Zerahemnah, took up the scalp from
off the ground, by the hair, and laid it upon the point of his
sword, and stretched it forth unto them. (Alma 20, pp.
346–347)

The evil Zerahemnah is dismembered twice in this passage, first
when his sword is broken at the hilt, and second when he is
scalped in a forme fruste of decapitation. Again, it is significant
that the two acts are not performed by Moroni himself, but instead by an unnamed surrogate, avoiding direct dismemberment
of the father.

One would think this action would be sufficient to end this
particular confrontation. However, when the Lamanites refuse to
submit, Moroni orders the Nephites to kill them:

And it came to pass that they began to slay them; yea, and the
Lamanites did contend with their swords and their mights.
But behold, their naked skins, and their bare heads, were exposed to the sharp swords of the Nephites; behold, they
were pierced and smitten; yea, and fell exceeding fast before
the swords of the Nephites; . . . (Alma 20, p. 347)

Could Joseph's imagery of the piercing and smiting of the naked
skins and bare heads reveal a clue to his own state of undress at
the fateful moment in his bedroom? One senses the entire matter
was as troubling for Joseph Smith, Jr., as for Zerahemnah.

There are at least two instances of another bizarre form of dismemberment ritual in *The Book of Mormon*—that of mass sword-
burying:

Now my best beloved brethren, since God hath taken away
our stains, and our swords have become bright, then let us
stain our swords no more with the blood of our brethren . . .
let us hide them away . . . we will bury them deep in the

earth, that they may be kept bright, as a testimony that we
have never used them, at the last day.

They took their swords, and all the weapons which were
used for the shedding of man's blood, and they did bury
them up deep in the earth; . . .

And it came to pass that when the people saw that [the La-
manites] were coming against them, they . . . prostrated
themselves before them to the earth . . . and thus they were
in this attitude, when the Lamanites began to fall upon
them, and began to slay them with the sword; and thus,
without meeting any resistance, they did slay a thousand
and five of them. (Alma 14, pp. 291–293)

There are several possible interpretations of this passage, all
sharing a common theme. Is it merely another fantasy reenactment of a punishing sword assault against powerless prostrate
victims as in the author's childhood? Is it a wish-fulfillment fantasy
that blood be washed from all knives that have done evil acts, and
that they be permanently hidden so they will not return "one
more time?" Is it a fantasy of punishment against those who have
so cruelly misused their knives in creating pain? Or does this passage suggest a boy's guilt over misusing his own "sword" for forbidden purposes? Is it thereby his promise never to do it again
that is symbolized in the passage by his pledge to bury it deep into
the earth so that he can never again perform the shameful act with
it? The passivity and powerlessness with which the punishment is
received in the prostrate position, the metaphor of shed blood,
and the ever-recurring theme of atonement for the sin specifically
recall the trauma once again.

The ritual is repeated an additional time:

And ye know also that they have buried their weapons of
war, and they fear to take them up, lest by any means they
shall sin; yea, ye can see that they fear to sin; for behold, they
will suffer themselves that they be trodden down and slain
by their enemies, and will not lift their swords against them.
(Helaman 5, p. 448)

Again, two themes are intertwined: one portraying the swords as amputation knives, and the other depicting the act of wielding the "sword" as the punishable "sin" of eroticism. The latter suggests that he will bury that weapon—will not lift his sword—and would rather be trodden down and slain by his enemies than sin again. Perhaps it would be better that the offensive thing be cut off and buried in the ground. The reenactments mirror the inseparable link in Joseph's own mind between eroticism and the imminent threat of violence.

Adoption Fantasy

Reference has been made to Joseph Smith, Jr.'s fondness for linking himself ancestrally, through the *The Book of Mormon* Jesus, to Joseph of the Old Testament. Such an assumption of noble parentage appears to suggest the presence of the well-known "adoption fantasy." Joseph Smith, Jr. thereby declares that he is not of humble background at all, but instead is of the most noble birth, by adopting himself into a Hebraic family of biblical greatness.

The adoption fantasy is surprisingly widespread among children. This fantasy imagines the parent, especially the boy's father, to be only a stepfather. The boy fantasizes instead that his true father is exalted and distinguished, unlike the one who claims to be his father and toward whom his aggressive and loathsome feelings demand vengeance. This fantasy says, in effect, "I am no longer your son nor your slave because someone else is my father." This dynamic is occasionally seen in adolescent boys who may actually change their given names (26).[6]

In Joseph Smith, Jr.'s case, however, the adoption fantasy carries an interesting twist. Rather than rejecting his biological father

---

[6] Maynard Solomon points out, for example, that Ludwig van Beethoven's lifetime mania to change the reality of his birthdate from 1770 to 1772 was an expression of this fantasy in an attempt to come to terms with repressed anger over an unhappy childhood at the hands of his father's irresponsibility, dishonesty, and alcoholism (27).

outright as is usually the case, Joseph, Jr. instead demonstrates his ambivalence by identifying positively through the inclusion of his father in the adoption fantasy. But he is relegated to the passive, lesser role of "father of the hero."

Often the form taken by "adoption" in *The Book of Mormon* is a sort of transfiguration of individuals or groups. In the early pages of the book, an angel prophesies to Nephi of the future in frontier America: "And it shall come to pass, that if the Gentiles shall hearken unto the Lamb of God . . . they shall be numbered among the House of Israel" (I Nephi 3, p. 32). In other words, those who believe that *The Book of Mormon* is divine will be adopted into Judaism under the aegis of the book's author (Lamb of God). In the same vein, and taking a leaf from Ethan Smith regarding the duty of white Americans to inform the Indians of their Hebraic ancestry, Joseph has Nephi's brother Jacob say, "I will afflict thy seed [the American Indians] by the hand of the Gentiles . . . that [the Gentiles] shall be like unto a father to them; wherefore, the Gentiles shall be blessed and numbered among the House of Israel" (II Nephi 7, p. 85).

In addition to the remote future, transfigurations in *The Book of Mormon* may be more immediate, taking place in the present through a mere change of mood:

> They were displeased with the conduct of their fathers, and they would no longer be called by the names of their fathers; therefore they took upon themselves the name of Nephi, that they might be called the children of Nephi, and be numbered among those which were called Nephites. (Mosiah 11, p. 208)

Again, it is specifically the shameful *fathers* who are rejected in favor of more suitable ancestors, as in Joseph's own adoption fantasy.

One sees the suggestion that family birth rank may also be subject to the "adoption fantasy." It is clear that the firstborn position was one that Joseph Smith, Jr. coveted within his own family. Alvin's death probably served, regardless of its pain to Joseph, as an act of wish-fulfillment of this fantasy. If he could not accept a middle-child status any more than he could accept being a son of the penurious Joseph Smith, Sr., he could merely fantasize himself into an adopted familial status more to his liking. After all, did he not deserve the position for having borne his father's name?

There is a kind of corollary to the firstborn theme in *The Book of Mormon* that suggests that firstborn sons may be unworthy of their birthrights. There are, for instance, many instances in which firstborn sons of rulers are passed over for the throne in favor of their younger brothers. In other circumstances the firstborn is chosen but is murdered or stripped of his throne by or on behalf of younger siblings, a different manner of literary expression of the same fantasy. Fratricidal stories abound throughout *The Book of Mormon*; reprieves, so universal in the case of attempted patricide, are few. Fratricidal events are seen as crimes of horror. As will be seen in Chapter 6, Joseph understood that horror well.

Role of Women

Because of the complexities of Joseph's own identification patterns, the male characters in *The Book of Mormon* show vastly greater character development than do the female characters. In fact, women play only bit parts in *The Book of Mormon,* but these roles are nonetheless very revealing of Joseph's attitudes toward women—an important prelude to his bold violations of societal conventions to be described in Chapter 7.

In fact, women seem to play only two roles in *The Book of Mormon*: faithful wife-mother and sexual object. Although such a bipolar view of women is commonly found in literature, it is nonetheless important to trace the origin and development of this theme in the life of Joseph Smith, Jr.

Women do not seem to be given much stature in *The Book of Mormon*. Although Nephi marries one of the daughters of Ishmael to raise the family who will become the Nephites of the story, his wife is never given the dignity of a name.

The traits of servility, subservience, and humility were for Joseph the attributes of women. It is a short distance from these phrases in *The Book of Mormon* to the prophecy he would shortly direct to his wife, Emma, in Harmony, Pennsylvania, in 1830:

> And the office of thy calling shall be for a comfort unto my servant Joseph Smith, jun., thy husband, in his afflictions, with consoling words, in the spirit of meekness . . .
>
> And thou needest not fear, for thy husband shall support thee from the church; for unto them is his calling . . .
>
> Continue in the spirit of meekness, and beware of pride. Let thy soul delight in thy husband, and the glory which shall come upon him. (28)

At times the subservient status of women is reinforced by the device of use of the phrase "women and children," implying a similar status of the two groups in society. It is never "men and women." Men, alone, stand as protagonists in all of the stories; on those rare occasions when women are mentioned as a group, children are invariably included as well.

But women had appeal to Joseph Smith, Jr. as sexual objects. When all was lost on the battlefield and massacre was at hand,

> [t]he king commanded them that all the men should leave their wives and their children, and flee before the Lamanites. Now there were many that would not leave them . . .
> . . . those that tarried with their wives and their children, caused that their fair daughters should stand forth and plead with the Lamanites, that they would not slay them. And . . . the Lamanites had compassion on them, for they were charmed with the beauty of their women; . . . (Mosiah 9, pp. 194–195)

In addition to men, women, and children, there appears to be a different social class called daughters. They have special traits of which Joseph takes special notice. On one occasion, for instance, the following occurred:

> Now there was a place in Shemlon, where the daughters of the Lamanites did gather themselves together for to sing, and to dance, and to make themselves merry. . . . having dis-

covered the daughters of the Lamanites, [Amulon's priests] laid and watched them; and when there were but few of them gathered together to dance, they came forth out of their secret places, and took them and carried them into the wilderness; yea, twenty and four of the daughters of the Lamanites they carried into the wilderness. (Mosiah 9, p. 196)

Battles ensue over this mass abduction and rape scene of Joseph's. But when Amulon's lascivious daughter-snatching priests are found and captured,

Amulon did plead with the Lamanites; and he also sent forth their wives, which was the daughters of the Lamanites, to plead with their brethren, that they should not destroy their husbands. And it came to pass that the Lamanites had compassion on Amulon and his brethren, and did not destroy them, because of their wives. (Mosiah 11, p. 204)

In other words, daughters may be ravished, and when they are, they will be appreciative and loyal to their ravishers. In Joseph's fantasy world order, daughters appear to have the status of grateful chattel.

There is a common denominator among these seemingly irreconcilable views of women: that of degradation, of regarding women as objects. It is this contempt that seems to propel Joseph's dual view of women as servants and sexual objects. They have well-defined roles and may never live on the plane of men. Much more of this attitude will be explored in Chapter 7 as it is played out in Joseph's own personal relationships with women.

Twelve

Before leaving *The Book of Mormon,* passing reference must be made to the number twelve, for it appears in numerous contexts. Twelve has special significance in the zodiacal tradition in which Joseph was raised, of course, but there may be other reasons for its special significance to him.

Jesus appointed twelve apostles, both in the New Testament

and in *The Book of Mormon* (III Nephi 5, p. 479). There were twelve Hebrew tribes, one for each of the sons of Jacob. There were twelve angels who followed the bright angel in Lehi's vision on the first pages of *The Book of Mormon*. The twelve apostles are designated to judge the twelve tribes of Israel. In a simple multiple, the evil priests of King Noah captured twenty-four daughters of the Lamanites in the abduction scene just described.

But beyond the biblical and astrological contexts, it is worth remembering that, as Joseph noted in his own account of his childhood illness, "[a]t one time eleven doctors came from Dartmouth Medical College, at Hanover, New Hampshire, for the purpose of amputation." With the addition of his father at the bedside to help with restraint, the number comes to twelve assailants for the ritualistic event that was the most significant event in his young life. As Terr points out, "Awareness of the presence of others is a powerful part of traumatic remembrance" (29). Twelve could hardly be other than a magical number in Joseph's troubled world.

The Book of Mormon, in its 590 pages, was a monumental effort for Joseph Smith, Jr. It was an impassioned expression of his conflicts as he dramatized them through the interplay of his many ancient characters. The book is probably no more nor less fictional than such Old Testament books as Genesis or Ruth, which it appears to emulate stylistically. However, the "validity" of *The Book of Mormon* lies not in literal truth any more than does *Hamlet,* for Joseph's creation certainly does not meet this criterion by any known historical evidence. It is "valid," however, as one person's metaphorical expression of the themes of guilt, punishment, redemption, grief, and the ambivalent relationship of man to "father" and "brother." To the extent that these expressions are universal in human experience and that meaningful communication occurs with the book's readers, *The Book of Mormon* is indeed as authentic a religious work as much of the more traditional body of "scriptural" writing. The fact that biographical study of the ancient authors of the metaphors contained in more familiar religious works is not usually possible should not obscure the similarity in expression of these most universal themes of human existence and the common threads in their origins. Nevertheless, understanding the uniquely personal origins of *The Book of Mormon* might be as important in understanding guilt, grief, shame, and father relationships as the study of traditional scripture itself.

Notes

1. Brodie F: *No Man Knows My History: The Life of Joseph Smith, the Mormon Prophet,* 2nd Edition. New York, Alfred A. Knopf, 1989, pp. 46–48.

2. Smith E: *View of the Hebrews; or the Ten Tribes of Israel in America,* 2nd Edition. Poultney, VT, 1825.

3. Persuitte D: *Joseph Smith and the Origins of The Book of Mormon.* Jefferson, NC, McFarland & Company, 1985, pp. 128–174.

4. Goodwin SH: *Additional Studies in Mormonism and Masonry.* Salt Lake City, Grand Lodge F. & A. M. of Utah, 1927.

5. Shengold L: *Soul Murder: The Effects of Childhood Abuse and Deprivation.* New Haven, CT, Yale University Press, 1989, pp. 5, 107.

6. Brodie F: *No Man Knows My History,* 2nd Edition, pp. 414–416; see p. 416.

7. Smith LM: *Biographical Sketches of Joseph Smith the Prophet and His Progenitors for Many Generations.* Liverpool, S. W. Richards, 1853 [reprinted New York, Arno Press, 1969], p. 73. Cited in Brodie F: *No Man Knows My History,* p. 414.

8. Freud S: "The Relationship of the Poet to Day-dreaming" (1908), in *Collected Papers,* Vol. 4. Translated and edited by Riviere J. New York, Basic Books, 1959, p. 173.

9. Howe ED: *Mormonism Unvailed.* Painesville, OH, 1834, p. 268.

10. Howe ED: *Mormonism Unvailed,* p. 269.

11. Bergmann T: "Observations of Children's Reactions to Motor Restraint." *The Nervous Child* 4:318–328, 1945.

12. *Doctrine and Covenants,* Section 50, vv. 41–43. Salt Lake City, Deseret News Company, 1880, p. 202.

13. Bettelheim B: *The Uses of Enchantment: The Meaning and Importance of Fairy Tales.* New York, Vintage Books, 1975, p. 159.

14. *Doctrine and Covenants,* Section 33, v. 1, p. 152.

15. Ibid., Section 19, vv. 15–18, 20, 22, pp. 118–119.

16. Ibid., Section 38, v. 4, p. 160.

17. Ibid., Section 29, vv. 18–19, p. 144.

18. Bettelheim B: *Symbolic Wounds: Puberty Rites and the Envious Male.* Glencoe, IL, Free Press, 1954, p. 128.

19. Ibid., p. 143.

20. Freud S: *The Interpretation of Dreams* (1900). Translated by Brill AA. New York, Macmillan Co., 1913, p. 246.

21. *Doctrine and Covenants,* Section 45, vv. 47–48, p. 187.

22. Ibid., Section 33, v. 7, p. 152.

23. Ibid., Section 121, v. 38, p. 424.

24. Ibid., Section 124, v. 99, p. 441.

25. Shengold L: *Soul Murder,* p. 107.

26. Gay P: *Freud for Historians.* New York, Oxford University Press, 1985, p. 197.

27. Solomon M: *Beethoven.* New York, Schirmer Books, 1977, pp. 3–6, 21–22.

28. *Doctrine and Covenants,* Section 25, vv. 5, 9, 14, respectively, p. 137. The 1880 and other later editions altered Joseph's phrase to read "support thee *in* the church" rather than his original "*from* the church."

29. Terr L: *Unchained Memories: True Stories of Traumatic Memories, Lost and Found.* New York, Basic Books, 1994, p. 35.

Chapter Six

His Brother's Keeper

*I*f *The Book of Mormon* story of Laban is the paradigm of Joseph Smith, Jr.'s inner conflicts concerning his father, the story of Jared seems to play a similar role with respect to a special sibling relationship. Like the story of Laban, that of Jared in the Book of Ether raises the curtain in the Old World as a family faces chaos and takes to the seashore. As noted in the previous chapter, the chaos in Jared's world is brought about when God decides to confound man's languages in punishment for constructing the Tower of Babel.

Jared is a unique character in *The Book of Mormon* for his lack of any identification with a father or any of the customary patriarchal lineage of other *The Book of Mormon* characters; instead, Jared's familial legitimacy is assured exclusively through a brother. In fact, to read *The Book of Mormon*'s Book of Ether, one might think "the brother of Jared" himself should have been given the hero's role for all of his marvelous

qualities and exploits. But in a book with some 300 named characters, this remarkable figure is never even given a name; his identity is always yoked to Jared's.

There is little question, however, that it is Jared—not his
brother—who is the extension in fantasy of the author's persona.
With the same first initial as Joseph's and a will that drives the plotline, Jared is the person through which Joseph's self-perceptions
are evident. Furthermore, although Jared himself is not described
in detail, the attributes ascribed to his brother are clearly *not*
those that Joseph has always used to describe the heroic character
of the book:

> And the brother of Jared, being a large and a mighty man,
> and being a man highly favored of the Lord; Jared his
> brother said unto him, Cry unto the Lord, that he will not
> confound us that we may not understand our words. And it
> came to pass that the brother of Jared did cry unto the Lord,
> and the Lord had compassion upon Jared; therefore he did
> not confound the language of Jared; and Jared and his
> brother were not confounded. (Ether 1, p. 539)

The mighty and protective ally, the powerful mediator with the
parent, the revered and idealized advocate—what small boy has
not on occasion viewed his older brother in such fashion?

As the story continues, Jared instructs his brother to ask the
Lord to take the two of them, along with their families and friends,
to "a land which is choice above all the earth." The Lord complies
and leads them to the seashore, where they live in preparation for
four years. Then the Lord returns in a cloud:

> And for the space of three hours did the Lord talk with the
> brother of Jared, and chastened him because he remem-
> bered not to call upon the name of the Lord. And the brother
> of Jared repented him of the evil which he had done, and did
> call upon the name of the Lord for his brethern which were
> with him. (Ether 1, p. 542)

Even the best brothers, one sees, are imperfect. They deserve pa-

rental scolding now and then for their effrontery. As in the story of
Laban, there is again at the seashore the need to rebuke a senior
male supporting character.

The Lord then gives instructions through the brother of Jared
for the construction of "barges."[1] But tightly closed cabins are
dark and frightening; one cannot face such terrifying enclosures
without light, for fear of the dark is very common in children after
surgical operations (1) (especially if Joseph had been blindfolded). The brother of Jared pleads for light for the barges and
climbs a mountain to smelt crystalline stones. He begs the Lord to
touch the stones with his finger to cause them "to shine in darkness, to give light unto men, women, and children [the inclusion
of children seems important here], that they might not cross the
great waters in darkness" (Ether 3, p. 548). In the encounter, the
brother of Jared is the first person to see Jesus Christ, is permitted
to see all of the future of humanity, is told to write all that he has
seen in an unreadable language, and is given two seer-stones that
should go with his writings for future translation "to the Gentiles." This brother is indeed an unusual figure of power and privilege whom the hero holds in awe.

However, when the time for succession of power arrives
among the growing clan in the Americas, the brother of Jared will
not be so fortunate despite what appears to be a clear birthright.
Always sensitive in his life to the issue of rank by birth order, Joseph Smith, Jr. gives strong clues that the brother of Jared is older
than Jared himself (e.g., larger, more assertive, twice as many children, and the first to perceive he was getting old). But when the
populace demands a king, the brother of Jared offers them the
combined pool of his own and Jared's sons from which to choose.
The people select Jared's brother's firstborn, who promptly de-
clines, as do all of his own brothers in turn. Then Jared's four sons
(as in the Smith family) are chosen in order; the youngest finally

---

[1] Although more traditional seafaring vessels with masts, sails, helm, and
rudder would have seemed more appropriate for ocean travel, one may
assume with some certainty that the imposing closed vessels being towed
through Palmyra along the Erie Canal following its completion in 1825 had
made the critical impression on the author.

accepts after the first three decline, and thus the mantle of leadership is passed from Jared's brother's line to Jared's. In the process it is twice affirmed that although birth order carries important rights, there are circumstances in which that privilege will be permitted to pass to younger brothers. It is an important principle for Joseph to legitimize.

The story of the brother of Jared is an unusual one in *The Book of Mormon* for its preponderance of the hero's worshipful feelings toward a brother. Thus, the story is not prototypical for the sibling rivalry that, as Brodie correctly points out (2), dominates the book. Why, then, has Joseph, Jr. given this story such prominence by its location in the prologue of the Old World, by the uniqueness of the brotherly relationship, and by the significance of a strong, righteous character who is not in the mold of "His Majesty the Ego," yet who sees God in the flesh and views prospectively all of human history? Could it be that Joseph was wishing to express some feelings about some very important and powerful individual in his life?

It would appear that "the brother of Jared" could symbolically represent one of only two persons: Alvin or Hyrum Smith. Although virtually nothing is known of the nature of the childhood relationships among the three oldest sons of Lucy and Joseph Smith, Sr., Alvin seems, by far, the more likely choice. Having died half-a-dozen years before the writing of *The Book of Mormon,* he would no longer have seemed an active rival for parental approval. Furthermore, the hostility felt by the family concerning the unkind words preached at the funeral could have evoked a spirit of defensiveness on his behalf. Alvin had held, in addition, clear title to the position of firstborn, a position Joseph evidently coveted.

If this supposition is correct, then the descriptions of the brother of Jared in *The Book of Mormon* may reveal important clues to Joseph's feelings toward Alvin. There is an obvious sense of hero worship and of his own inferiority in Joseph's description of the brother of Jared as "a large and a mighty man, and being a man highly favored of the Lord [read Father]." Near the end of *The Book of Mormon,* the Joseph Smith–like Moroni expresses the difference between the two characters:

> Behold, thou hast not made us mighty in writing like unto
> the brother of Jared, for thou madest him that the things
> which he wrote, were mighty even as thou art, unto the over-
> powering of man to read them . . . wherefore, when we
> write, we behold our weakness, and stumble because of the
> placing of our words; and I fear lest the Gentiles shall mock
> at our words . . . for the brother of Jared said unto the
> mountain Zerin, Remove, and it was removed. (Ether 5,
> pp. 564–565)

Of course, as Bettelheim points out in his sensitive study of fairy
tales (3), all children see grownups and older children as strong
and themselves as weak.

   Indeed, Joseph's own remembrance of Alvin carries the same
worshipful surrealism as that of the fictional Jared toward his
brother:

> Alvin . . . was the oldest, and the noblest of my father's fam-
> ily. He was one of the noblest of the sons of men . . . In him
> there was no guile. He lived without spot from the time he
> was a child. From the time of his birth, he never knew mirth.
> He was candid and sober and never would play; and minded
> his father, and mother, in toiling all day. He was one of the
> soberest of men and when he died the angel of the Lord vis-
> ited him in his last moments. (4)

The identity of the brother of Jared can hardly be in doubt.

   The plotline itself provides important evidence that it is Alvin
who is symbolized by the brother of Jared. By seeing Jesus Christ
in the flesh before Jesus' earthly birth, the brother of Jared plays
a kind of John the Baptist role as though he would foreshadow
a more important person. It is likely that Joseph, Jr. in his own
sense of self-grandeur saw Alvin in just such a light. (This analogy
may be more than coincidentally associated with the fate of *be-
heading,* by which John the Baptist was removed from the story at
the advent of Christ.) The fact that the brother of Jared receives
the two seer-stones (Urim and Thummim) from Jesus with instructions, in effect, to see that they are safely passed to Joseph
Smith, Jr., some 4,000 to 5,000 years hence is but a slightly differ-

ent way of expressing the same fantasy. This *passing of the torch* is
the subliminal message of the story of the brother of Jared. It is
seen both in the succession to leadership and power and in the
transfer of the stones.

Gleaning this cryptic message from *The Book of Mormon* demands that a much closer examination be undertaken of the likely
effect of Alvin's death on Joseph. Mention has already been made
in the previous chapter of the fact that Joseph attempted to join
the Baptist Church shortly after this tragic event. The family's anger toward the physician and toward the minister presiding at the
funeral has been described, with both reactions very possibly representing a collective effort by the family to deal with their own
frustration and shame over the event by projecting it outside the
family. The bizarre exhumation was carried out several months
later. Furthermore, the tone throughout the early portion of Lucy's
biography suggests that Alvin had in fact been the leader of the children and a special favorite of hers, and there is additional evidence
in support of Alvin's "chosen" position in his parents' eyes. The
Smith neighbors Orasmus Turner and J. H. Kennedy both quoted
the parents as saying that Alvin specifically was to be the one with
the special gifts. Other neighbors from Palmyra had identified Alvin
as a treasure-seeker and "seer" prior to his death (5).

It is likely that Joseph's adoption of the firstborn position as
Alvin's "replacement" may well have had another impetus as well.
Cain and Cain have described a frequent grief reaction in parents
over the loss of a favored child in which replacement of the dead
child is attempted through the parents' attempted substitution of
a surviving younger sibling (6). By this mechanism or any of its
variants, however, only a *pseudoresolution* of the mourning process is ever achieved because the intense bonds and yearnings for
the favored child are merely redirected toward a younger sibling.
When such en bloc transfer of affection and aspirations occurs,
truly successful mourning for the lost child is aborted, and sorrow
and depression may persist more or less indefinitely, with unnatu-
rally high expectations for the "substitute" child. This failure to
complete a healthy mourning process may adversely affect the
process for all members of the household. If this was the case for
Joseph, Jr. in the Smith household, the environment could easily

have reinforced the boy's craving for the firstborn position and have given it a sense of legitimacy alongside his more complex feelings over the loss.

At the time of Alvin's demise at age 25 (Joseph was then 17), all nine Smith children were apparently unmarried and still residing with their parents. It is a fair assumption that the internal family dynamics of the earlier stages of childhood persisted through this unceasing proximity to one another. If, as suggested previously, Joseph felt from his early childhood both admiration and envy for his big brother, these feelings should not have been much altered in such tight living quarters during Joseph's advancement into adolescence.

If nothing were known other than this bare skeleton of knowledge about the Smith family's interpersonal dynamics, it would be difficult to speculate on Joseph's true emotions at this difficult time. However, as was done in the case with children undergoing surgical operations and other emotional trauma, it is possible to turn to contemporary psychiatric studies to see how other children have responded to similar events.

Among several studies that have addressed the issue of sibling death, one by Cain and colleagues is particularly instructive (7). The principal reaction to sibling death described in this study was overwhelming guilt,

> with the guilt still consciously active five years or more after the sibling's death. Such children felt responsible for the death, sporadically insisted it was all their fault, felt they should have died too, or should have died *instead* of the dead sibling . . . They mulled over and over the nasty things they had thought, felt, said or done to the dead sibling, and became all the guiltier. They also tried to recall the good things they had done, the ways they had protected the dead sibling, and so on. The guilt was variously handled by each child in accord with his unique personality structure . . . (8)

Joseph Smith, Jr. had to have integrated Alvin's death through his own preexisting filters of guilt, punishment, narcissism, and fantasy.

Cain et al. go on to state:

> Where either the realities or the aggressive fantasies sur-
> rounding the death left the remaining sibling struggling
> with intense guilt, the child typically grew extremely fearful
> of losing control of his anger and experienced himself as
> a monster and potential killer. He attempted various identi-
> fications which all cried out that he was in no way aggressive
> or capable of such behavior, generally withdrew and per-
> ceived situations in which he might do *anything* wrong as
> reverberating of the past wrongdoing, the "killing." (9)

With this in mind, it is worth noting the numerous instances
in *The Book of Mormon* in which the hero of the moment scolds
the multitude for their many transgressions, setting himself
apart in his own conduct. The hero customarily runs down a litany of specific evil acts in these instances, and at the head of the
list, more often than not, is murder (e.g., ". . . and that they
might be convinced that they were all brethren, and that they
had not ought to murder, nor to plunder, nor to steal, nor to
commit adultery, nor to commit any manner of wickedness").
There was no known murder in the personal experience of Joseph Smith, Jr., if one disregards the incident of the stray bullet
near the house mentioned earlier in this chapter. The 1826 murder of William Morgan, the Freemason, was a popular, short-
lived cause in upstate New York but scarcely seems to be a candi-
date for this degree of preeminence among the list of evils in *The
Book of Mormon*. While it seems extremely unlikely that Joseph,
Jr. participated in any way in the intra-abdominal catastrophe
that caused Alvin's death, it is quite permissible to postulate that
he *believed* he had. And in so doing, he had "overthrown" the
firstborn.

If, in fact, one makes the assumption that Joseph believed
himself, by whatever twist of fantasy, to have been responsible
in some manner for Alvin's death, some previously puzzling items
in the historical record begin to make sense for the first time. In
Joseph's 1826 trial in Bainbridge, New York, for instance, Jonathan Thompson, in his testimony cited in Chapter 4, described

Joseph's dissociative, stone-staring trance in leading a dig for a chest of money:

> After digging several feet, struck upon something sounding like a board or plank. Prisoner would not look again, pretending that he was alarmed the last time that he looked, on account of the circumstances relating to the trunk being buried came all fresh to his mind; that the last time that he looked he discovered distinctly the two Indians who buried the trunk; that a quarrel ensued between them, and that one of said Indians was killed by the other, and thrown in the hole beside of the trunk, to guard it, as he supposed. (10)

What if Joseph was, in fact, perhaps not merely "pretending that he was alarmed," as Thompson had presumed, but was instead reacting legitimately to a most frightening flashback of a fratricidal fantasy that the dig had brought to mind? Such late-adolescent flashbacks, as in the case of troubled combat veterans, are invariably associated with just the sort of cold, sweaty, panicky "tape-review" experiences at just the wrong moment of recognition, as Thompson described. If so, what could have been the relationship between the excavation of a trunk and the memory of Alvin's death? And why should the sound of impact of a shovel on a buried board have provoked Joseph into such a terrifying and paralyzing flashback?

If all Mormon historical orthodoxy concerning this series of events may be put aside, some new speculations may be helpful in answering these questions. Cain et al.'s study of sibling death suggests that a child who believes himself or herself to have been the monstrous killer of a sibling will find his or her guilt magnified by any additional family reactions that develop from that death. If it is recalled that Joseph, Sr. arranged a grotesque exhumation of Alvin's body several months after the burial and then published his strange notice in the local newspaper, it might be asked if this event in fact brought Joseph, Jr.'s guilt to the breaking point through his ghastly observation of the putrid spectacle of his brother's rotting corpse, the rekindled grief of his parents, and the perceived ridicule toward himself of much of the community. After all, this would apparently have been the only moment in his life when a treasure dig actually found a box with its intended contents! And just as a car's backfire may spark a flashback in an infantry veteran, the sound of a shovel on a plank could have been a most appropriate "trigger" for Joseph if this notion is correct. What individual with a sense for the erotic excitement of the treasure hunt would not have been haunted by such a grotesque and perverse reality at the end of the shovel?

It is inconceivable that Joseph, Jr. would not have attended the exhumation in view of its importance to family traditions, though his father's newspaper account refers only to "some of my neighbors" in attendance. But since Joseph, Jr. appears never to have made any direct reference to having seen the corpse, his subsequent apparent repetitions of the event in fantasy suggest that this event, too, was probably not available to conscious memory. Terr reports that children who merely hear about an event of horror have no accompanying behavioral symptoms: "A horrifying tale alone does not cause the mind to malfunction. Even if the tale is inserted by the most adept of brainwashers, the child will exhibit no symptoms to go along with the 'memory'" (11).

It is usually accepted at face value by historians of Mormonism that the motivation for the exhumation was in some way related to a cruel practical joke. Either pranksters were poking fun at the digging practices of Joseph, Jr. and his father by spreading rumors of grave robbing, or the pranksters were preying on Joseph's reported need to exhibit a part of Alvin's body in order to obtain his treasure since he had supposedly been instructed by the angel Moroni a year previously to return in a year with Alvin as his intercessor. Hence, the proximity of the newspaper account on September 25, 1824, to the date of the alleged second annual visit to Hill Cumorah on September 22, 1824.

But annual ritualistic pilgrimages to a special place are typical of a well-known pattern of repetitive behavior performed in response to a stressful event. Such defenses are referred to as "anniversary reactions." These anniversaries of painful events may be marked by unusual behavioral rituals that often can be understood only by uncovering the nature of the event that they in some way "memorialize" (12). The best known are in relation to deathdays, anniversaries of assaults or rapes or suicides, or other fixed dates. Behavior on these occasions may be ritualistic and driven by powerful emotions as a defense against the pain of the original event. As such, the *content* of the behavior itself may often give clues to the identity of the memorialized event (13).

As an alternative explanation, therefore, it is possible that the traditional view of the visits to the hill as a prospective series of annual events may in fact be exactly the opposite: an elaborate retrospective fantasy ritual based on the anniversary of the original wrenching exhumation of Alvin's body on September 25, 1824. As such, all but the last of the five annual "visits" to Hill Cumorah did not occur at all, but were instead merely elaborate annual fantasies generated out of the horror of the exhumation and of Joseph's guilt over his imagined complicity in Alvin's death.

In fact, of all the early descriptions about Joseph's acquisition of the plates, only the sanctifying accounts of Joseph's aged mother and two aged siblings carry any firsthand corroboration of any actual visits at all to Hill Cumorah before the final one in September 1827, and these make no reference to any annual visits in 1824, 1825, or 1826. Younger brother William was 72 years old when he recalled the events of his teens. In his version there is even an 1823 angelic foretelling of the four-year delay before Joseph may receive the plates, directly contradicting Joseph's own account, but making no reference to annual visits (14, 15). Lucy's description confirms that none of the family was aware of any annual visits to the hill or the time he would obtain the plates (16). At age 72, Joseph's younger sister, Katharine, made reference to his going "frequently to the hill" and reporting his finds to the family, apparently contradicting both Emma and William but still making no reference to annual September 22 events (17).

All other allusions to pre-1827 visits to Hill Cumorah in the published record are secondhand accounts attributed retrospectively to Joseph or to his parents from the year 1827 or thereafter. These accounts include those of Willard Chase (first briefed by Joseph Smith, Sr. in June 1827) (18), Benjamin Saunders (most likely briefed by Joseph Smith, Jr. after September 1827, according to Quinn) (19), Joseph Knight (briefed apparently by Joseph Smith, Jr. in time for him to be present at the Smith home on September 22, 1827, but there is no evidence that Knight knew anything of prior visits to the hill except what Joseph had narrated retrospectively to him) (20), Martin Harris (formally briefed with an accompanying request for financial support by Joseph Smith, Jr. in the fall of 1827) (21), Henry Harris (briefed by Joseph Smith, Jr. after September 1827) (22), and Oliver Cowdery (1828). The fact that Lucy's account parallels Joseph's own written narration of piety for this period and contains none of the important but embarrassing money-digging activities of the period from 1823 to 1827 further supports the historiographic view that her account, as filtered through her literary collaborators, drew heavily on Joseph's own retrospective narrative in order to build a coherent framework of early history as a sort of institutional polemic. This distortion on the part of Lucy and her collaborators is further substantiated by her and her sons Hyrum and Samuel having been in reality active members of the Palmyra Presbyterian Church from 1820 until about September 1828, a fact excluded from her narrative (23).

However, Jonathan Thompson's sworn testimony in the 1826 trial is suggestive evidence in psychoanalytic terms that Joseph had a dissociated memory of the exhumation event that was playing a role in his fantasies during the period dating back at least to the 1825 treasure-digging episode itself. The fantasy of one Indian killing another and burying him with a trunk, the triggering of a flashback of that fantasy by the sound of a shovel against something like a board of a trunk, and the panicky terror associated with that sudden recall of the fantasy are difficult to ignore, especially as narrated by a sworn, disinterested witness who had been present at the event itself. In this sense, one can make an argument that there is greater artifactual evidence for a complex ritual of fantasy surrounding Alvin's exhumation than for any actual September visits to the hill before 1827.

Thus, if this speculation about the true significance to Joseph of Alvin's exhumation is correct, the elaborate story of the annual treasure-seeking visits to the hill seems to have been backdated by Joseph to the first anniversary *before* the exhumation, and thus the true inciting event for the anniversary reaction would be obscured. Joseph thus incorporated Alvin into the story, assuaging his guilt by making Alvin a central partner in obtaining the plates—much the same message as in the story of the brother of Jared.

It will be helpful to review what Joseph retrospectively claimed to have occurred on these successive anniversaries during the four years before 1827. On September 22, 1823, the story begins as the angel strikes Joseph and tells him he may not have the plates until he returns in one year with his oldest brother. On September 22, 1824, as Joseph evolved the story, the plates would certainly have been given to him had Alvin not died. Instead, Joseph would be punished again on this occasion and asked to find an Alvin-substitute. On September 22, 1825, a fellow treasure-digger, Samuel Lawrence, is offered (though there is only a single account of this) with no success. On September 22, 1826, Joseph reports that he is told that he must find and bring a suitable Alvin-substitute the following year or he will *never* obtain the plates.

If all of these visits are recast as pure fantasy, retrospective from 1827, there seems to be a hidden theme: the central role of Alvin in the quest. When Joseph is unable to produce his eldest brother in 1824, it is as though he is being punished for Alvin's absence by having the plates withheld. A punishment fantasy would be consistent with a sense of guilt on Joseph's part over in some way his causing Alvin's absence and usurping the "firstborn" role. The fantasied request by the treasure guardian for an Alvin-substitute makes Alvin a necessary partner in the creation of *The Book of Mormon*. Through this construction of fantasy, Joseph could assuage his own lingering guilt over his anguished, imagined complicity in his brother's death. The selection of Samuel Lawrence as an Alvin-substitute possibly suggests that Joseph identified Alvin at some level as a comrade, like Lawrence himself, in the money-digging fellowship. Indeed, Alvin is no bit player in this treasure quest; he is the prime mover of the event. Inscribed on the inside cover of *Manuscript History of the Church,* Book A-1, is Joseph's notation, "In Memory of Alvin Smith, Died the 19th Day of November, In the 25th year of his age year 1823" (24).[2]

---

[2] The original note incorrectly read "1824," with the 4 overwritten with a 3, the correct digit, in different ink sometime later. This leads to the interesting speculation of another "Freudian slip" on Joseph's part—that

In the meantime, Joseph had become enamored of Emma Hale and had eloped with her in January 1827.[3] In 1827, when the September 22 anniversary in Joseph's story arrived, Joseph's apparent achievement of an intimate relationship had made the time propitious for consummating his treasure-search. The Fraiberg schema of treasure-seeking as a sexual fantasy therefore continues to serve as an important framework for the fantasies.

However, the puzzling odyssey of anniversary visits seems to occur outside and independently of the underlying sexual theme of the story. On some level, Joseph's tale of repeated annual delays may be a clue to his perception that he was not yet old enough to take on the mantle of a brother whose memory was permanently cast in his midtwenties, Alvin's age when he died. Yet, the complex elaboration of the retrospective fantasy of all those repeated annual trips up the hill makes sense only through Joseph's apparent need to include Alvin as his essential partner in the story for having somehow cheated Alvin out of his birthright.

Perhaps the final confirmation that this is the case is provided by the ultimate role played by Emma as Joseph's key to unlocking the treasure-guardian's resistance to releasing the plates. On some level of consciousness Joseph might have perceived that his new wife was not herself the substitute but merely the mechanism by which he could procreate his own Alvin-substitute through the sexuality of the treasure quest. It will be remembered that Joseph's deformed son was born nine to ten months after the acquisition

---

perhaps it was indeed the horrid 1824 exhumation through which he was haunted by his lost brother, and not Alvin's actual 1823 demise. In fact, Joseph made exactly the same slip on a second occasion in referring to his 1827 visit to Hill Cumorah as the "fourth year" rather than the fifth (see Jessee DC: *The Personal Writings of Joseph Smith*. Salt Lake City, Deseret Book Company, 1984, p. 77). The slip occurred even a third time, in Joseph's *Manuscript History of the Church* (Book A-1, p. 7).

[3] Could the hastiness of this marriage have been itself an expression of sibling rivalry, since his remaining older brother, Hyrum, had become the first in the family to marry just two months previously? Did such an adultlike action on the part of his remaining older sibling threaten Joseph, Jr.'s own claim to Alvin's mantle of firstborn?

of his treasure and that Joseph had indicated to Isaac Hale and others during the pregnancy that a child would be the first to view the plates. Sophia Lewis quoted Joseph as saying "the Book of Plates could not be opened under penalty of death by any other person but his (Smith's) first-born, which was to be a male" (25). Joshua M'Kune swore that "Joseph Smith, Jr. told him that (Smith's) first-born child was to translate the characters, and heiroglyphics, upon the Plates into our language at the age of three years" (26). But of far greater significance, Willard Chase had indicated that Martin Harris "reported that the Prophet's wife, in the month of June following would be delivered of a male child that would be able when two years old to translate the Gold Bible" (27)—a nine-month prediction that *absolutely* establishes Joseph's fantasy of the treasure search as a symbol of sexual consummation and conception. If Joseph, Jr. and Emma were like most excited first-time parents-to-be, they would have planned months in advance for the name to be given to the new member of the family. Though tiny *Alvin* lived only three hours, he yet probably served his grieving daddy by helping him to assuage a burden of guilt and sadness.

This hypothesis further helps to explain Joseph's otherwise puzzling personal need to elaborate a bizarre and complicated story for the seemingly straightforward task of climbing a hill and carrying down the plates. Although treasure-seeking fantasies invariably require some twists of intrigue by the hero to get his prize away from the treasure's paternal guardian, it appears to have been from the dissociated corners of Joseph's own mind that the unique specifics of these convoluted fantasies became embodied in this particular anniversary ritual. From an infinity of available plotlines he apparently elaborated this highly unusual one for a special reason.

Joseph must have had an additional pragmatic reason to elaborate this particular tale, since he would have known that the story would not have meshed well with his known scandalous money-digging activities during the four years before 1827. Because the existing historical record from sources outside the Smith family does not corroborate much piety on the part of Joseph or the family before 1827, it has been difficult for many historians to take seriously the scenario of four years of a superstitious lifestyle of commerce in black magic and neighborhood contempt alongside a parallel commitment of deep humility, devout religious obedience, and self-denial. The difficulty has lain not in the acceptance of a religious "conversion" by Joseph, but rather in the embracing of the notion of the coexistence of incompatibly disparate lifestyles simultaneously during the four years between 1823 and 1827.

Joseph was troubled by hidden memories and feelings on a specific date in September each year after the 1824 exhumation, and it appears that he may have dealt with them characteristically in metaphor and fantasy. The coloration with religious overtones seems to have been a kind of afterthought, introduced in 1827, in keeping with the entire evolution of the concept of *The Book of Mormon,* especially as it apparently became necessary for Joseph to obscure the embarrassing aspects of his money-digging activities. But a less-than-conscious fantasy ritual, played out in his mind on each anniversary of Alvin's exhumation and deliberately redressed in 1827 in religious clothing, seems a more plausible explanation for Joseph's colorful story than does the allegation of a theophany in September 1823 and a series of annual interviews with an angel. The clues provided by the story of the brother of Jared make this hypothesis a plausible one. There may be a better explanation that does not include human toads, angels, and bleeding ghosts, but it is not readily apparent. The 1823 Second Vision seems a doubtful event.

But if this was the case, one might ask, why wouldn't Joseph have used the *actual* date of the exhumation, September 25, instead of September 22, three days earlier, for the anniversary? Was he trying to camouflage the nature of the true origin of the anniversary since the notice in the newspaper had been published in several editions and was on the public record? In fact, there was no deception whatsoever. A review of calendar tables discloses that September 25, 1824, the date of the hideous exhumation, fell on the fourth Saturday of the month. Since, as has already been described, Joseph appears to have formalized this anniversary ritual with his plan for a history of the Moundbuilders only in 1827, backdating it annually from that time, it is specifically 1827 that would have required the formal announcement of an actual date for the special occurrence. Not surprisingly, the fourth Saturday of the month in 1827 did indeed fall on the September 22, the true anniversary of Joseph's pain. It was at the end of the week's labors that his father had unearthed Alvin's decaying corpse. Although his father had declared his announcement by its date in the month for publication in the local newspaper, it is likely that Joseph, Jr.'s dissociated memories of the awful event were associated with the week's end, for activities at the end of the week, then as now, were different from the monotonous activities of midweek. The fourth Saturday of September was the date of the exhumation and the date of Joseph, Jr.'s annual fantasies of bereavement. The numerical day of the month is irrelevant. And the fourth Saturday is the same date Joseph would climb the hill to obtain a legacy from the brother for whom he so deeply grieved—the sight of whose rotting corpse still haunted him. Mere coincidence in dates seems less likely.

How then to account for the earliest year of backdating—the placement of the inciting Second Vision into 1823 rather than 1824, when the exhumation occurred? Was this a conscious deception by Joseph designed to cover up the scent of the trail? It is doubtful. As noted in Chapter 3, Terr has frequently observed skewing of time in traumatized children—the way they commonly reorder time sequences around the traumatic event. In the process such children typically develop a pattern of inventing "omens" by placing events that postdate the trauma into positions *before* the trauma in their mind's temporal order. This second dreadful trauma in Joseph's life—the horror-laden exhumation of the putrefying corpse of a loved sibling—occurred against the background of a psyche already sufficiently crippled by a previous brutal childhood trauma that there was a preformed dissociated pattern for dealing with shocking events. In this type of emotionally charged setting, in which the mind deceives itself far more often than it deceives others, time does funny things. The entire Second Vision fantasy, with its elaborate anniversary pattern of repetition, affirms the remarkable dimension to which time-skew and repetitive dreaming may be elaborated in the inner struggle with a traumatic event. The individual impacts of the two sequential traumas in Joseph's life were thus multiplied in the creation of a truly elaborate and seductive story. There was no "deception." The dissociated part of Joseph's mind played it out in the way it could best ease his pain and guilt.

A review of the major repetitive themes in the content of this anniversary reaction points toward the exhumation as the inciting event. The first piece of evidence is the identical date—the fourth Saturday in September—for the event and its anniversaries. The second is the basic plotline of unearthing a box with a treasure of immense value that could be viewed but not taken. The third is the recurring theme of the annual need to produce a substitute for Alvin, with Joseph placing his brother as the key to the treasure and the pivotal character in the story. The fourth is the repetition of punishment for some shortcoming at each visit—being knocked to the ground, being forbidden to take away the treasure that one could see and hold but not possess—as though he felt guilt for some ill-defined but unspeakable act. Again, Joseph chose guilt over shame as he elaborated a fantasy of punishment rather than to accept the feeling of random powerlessness at the death of a sibling.

What, then, really *did* happen on the fourth Saturday of September in 1825 and 1826, the two years that are not accounted for (since 1823 was a backdated fantasy and 1824 was the actual year of the exhumation)? Did Joseph stand on those dates at Alvin's grave with bereavement fantasies and hideous memories of the rotting corpse flooding over him? Did he beg his departed brother's forgiveness for not being the affectionate little brother he should have been or for not having saved his life? Did his mind, in a posttraumatic convulsion to expunge the horrible visage of the rotting corpse, spin forth a wishful hallucination of a radiant brother wearing a "loose robe of most exquisite whiteness"—fragments of daydream material that would be elaborated into what he came to call his "Second Vision," or perhaps his "First," or both? Perhaps on one of those two days, when the bereavement fantasies were flooding over him most strongly, he took a walk up a nearby hill—perhaps with Samuel Lawrence. Did he pause near a treasure-digging site or recall Alvin's presence on past digs? One suspects that those September anniversaries in 1825 and

1826—the silent Saturdays—were seminal moments for the elaboration of that daydream material. But one can only imagine.

It would be convenient if a ready explanation were apparent for Joseph, Sr.'s decision to exhume Alvin's body in the first place, but this remains the unsolved mystery. Both of the customary explanations outlined on p. 138 share the feature that Alvin's father was reacting rationally to external events, though any connection to a nonexistent annual encounter with an angel may be ruled out. If one additional explanation may be ventured, it is worth considering that the initiative may have been primary with Joseph, Sr., and perhaps without any rational basis whatever. Simple logic would suggest that mere inspection of the ground over the ten-month-old grave would have been sufficient to determine whether a violation had occurred, especially if such were recent. It seems more plausible that in his tortured grief, the father might have initiated the event himself in order to see Alvin again or to try to resurrect him or to commune with him in some way through the intricacies of the magic arts, as a main focus of Joseph Sr.'s life seems to have been ritualistically digging in the ground for lost treasures of spirits. If so, the reasons implied in his newspaper announcement were then merely *defensive rationalizations* of his action, as he would have had need preemptively to protect himself against prosecution for violating a grave, a felony offense for which, in 1824, he could have been incarcerated in the New York state prison for five years (28).

Having carried the hypothesis about Joseph, Jr. and Alvin's death this far, however, we could ask why not to carry it one step further to its logical conclusion? The short Book of Ether itself—the entire "afterthought" of the story of the Jaredites, separated in time from the main body of the story by 2,400 years—must be seen as Joseph's independent tribute to Alvin. Joseph could have created "the brother of Alma," "the brother of Mosiah," or "the brother of Lamoni" to accomplish the same literary end in the principal body of the story of Lehi's family, but it would not have been sufficiently ennobling. The issue of Alvin's death was particularly troubling to Joseph and probably occupied nearly as great a place in the brooding dissociated corners of his mind as did the issue represented by the story of Laban. It therefore needed to be granted an equivalent stature in *The Book of Mormon* by placing it, too, in the prologue of the Old World. But since there was no room for a character as exalted as Alvin in the well-developed story of Lehi's family, a second exodus had to be created. The Book of Ether could thus allow Joseph an uncluttered development of his eulogy to Alvin in its initial twelve pages, following which he could rapidly accelerate the pace of the rest of the story. The rise and annihilation of an entire civilization occur in the remaining twenty-three pages of the Book of Ether, perhaps an indication that the portion of the story extolling the brother of Jared was the reason Joseph had written this particular book in the first place. Thus it would seem that the appearance of this highly unusual character in *The Book of Mormon,* supremely honored as was Yahweh by having a name so mighty that it could not be spoken, is the testimony of Joseph's anguish over his lost brother.

But the testimony would not be limited to *The Book of Mormon,* though finding cryptic allusions to Alvin's death in the biographical record is not so easy as seeking allusions to Joseph's childhood operation. The latter seem to have emerged metaphorically from a large number of Joseph's elaborate rituals, innovations, writings, and impassioned speeches. But as the apparent guilt over Alvin's death needed assuaging, disguised representations of this deeply personal conflict must also be sought.

A reasonable place to start is the First Vision—the early angelic visitation that Joseph claimed to be the prime mover of his prophetic activity. Brodie has pointed out that this theophany, which supposedly occurred in 1820 when Joseph was 14 years of age, was never mentioned in any historical source until 1838 when Joseph began his elaborate autobiography. The fact that all of the numerous accounts given by him and his family members and apologists before 1838 failed to mention the First Vision led Brodie to question the authenticity of Joseph's claim to the event at all except perhaps as "the elaboration of some half-remembered dream stimulated by the early revival excitement," or, alternatively, "sheer invention, created some time after 1830 when the need arose for a magnificent tradition to cancel out the stories of his fortune-telling and money-digging" (29).

But whenever it occurred—or whether it was a dream, a daydream, or an awake backdated composition—the description has the same authorship. The following is an example of the precise visual detail in Joseph's description:

> I kneeled down and began to offer up the desires of my heart to God. I had scarcely done so, when immediately I was seized upon by some power which entirely overcame me, and had such an astonishing influence over me as to bind my tongue so that I could not speak. Thick darkness gathered around me, and it seemed to me for a time as if I were doomed to sudden destruction. . . . I saw a pillar of light exactly over my head, above the brightness of the sun, which descended gradually until it fell upon me. It no sooner appeared than I found myself delivered from the enemy which held me bound. When the light rested upon me I saw two personages, whose brightness and glory defy all description, standing above me in the air. One of them spake unto me, calling me by name, and said—pointing to the other—"This is my beloved son, hear him." . . . I asked the personages who stood above me in the light, which of all the sects was right—and which I should join. I was answered that I must join none of them, for they were all wrong, and the personage who addressed me said that all their creeds were an abomination in His sight. . . . He again forbade me to join with any of them: and many other things did he say unto me, which I cannot write at this time. When I came to myself again, I found myself lying on my back, looking up into heaven . . . (30)

Leaving aside the historical record that documents Joseph's two subsequent actions in joining local churches, a curious fact of the "dream content" stands out. There is not one father-image but *two,* and they are related to each other as father and son. The father seems to "legitimize" the son's authority by introducing him, and the son takes up the dialogue to instruct Joseph in ways that will lead to his privileged uniqueness as prophet.

This scenario, of course, is a variation of the same message that was expressed with the brother of Jared in the Book of Ether. It is the image of a benevolent older brother, bestowed with the explicit imprimatur of the father, who instructs, intercedes, and passes a mantle of leadership to Joseph. The First Vision seems in this respect to be as much of a tribute to Alvin (and perhaps as much a balm to Joseph's lingering feelings over Alvin's death) as is the Book of Ether. This, if true, would provide further support to Brodie's view of a backdating of the doubtful event, since Alvin's death did not occur until Joseph was 17 years of age, in 1823, three years after the alleged date of the first theophany. Again, Terr's observations of posttraumatic time-skew and "omens" (see Chapter 3) appear relevant in this instance. As described with the Second Vision, the backdating of the First Vision appears to have been just such a posttraumatic reordering of time sequence and likely not a conscious deception.

But what is to be made of the content of the Second Vision, that event that ostensibly launched the treasure quest to *The Book of Mormon*? As Joseph described it, with much visual detail, in his personal history:

> On the evening of the above-mentioned twenty-first of September, after I had retired to my bed for the night, . . . I discovered a light appearing in my room, which continued to increase until the room was lighter than at noonday, when immediately a personage appeared at my bedside, standing in the air, for his feet did not touch the floor. He had on a loose robe of most exquisite whiteness. It was a whiteness beyond anything earthly I had ever seen; nor do I believe that any earthly thing could be made to appear so exceedingly white and brilliant. His hands were naked and his arms also, a little above the wrist, so, also were his feet naked, as were his legs, a little above the ankles. His head and neck were also bare. I could discover that he had no other clothing on but this robe, as it was open, so that I could see into his bosom. Not only was his robe exceedingly white, but his whole person was glorious beyond description, and his countenance truly like lightning. The room was exceedingly light, but not so very bright as immediately around his per-

son. . . . He called me by name, and said unto me that he was a messenger sent from the presence of God to me and that his name was Nephi; . . . He said there was a book deposited, written upon gold plates giving an account of the former inhabitants of this continent, and the sources from whence they sprang. He also said that the fullness of the everlasting Gospel was contained in it, as delivered by the Savior to the ancient inhabitants; also that there were two stones in silver bows—and these stones, fastened to a breastplate, constituted what is called the Urim and Thummim—deposited with the plates; and the possession and use of these stones were what constituted seers in ancient or former times. (31)

After some scripture is quoted, the Second Vision narrative continues:

While he was conversing with me about the plates, the vision was opened to my mind that I could see the place where the plates were deposited, and that so clearly and distinctly that I knew the place again when I visited it.

After this communication, I saw the light in the room began to gather immediately around the person of him who had been speaking to me, and it continued to do so, until the room was again left dark, except just around me, when instantly I saw, as it were, a conduit open right up into heaven, and he ascended until he entirely disappeared. (32)

Second and third identical visits follow, which Joseph describes with the same vivid visual details.[4] Since it is by then morning in Joseph's narrative, he arises and goes to the fields but is sent home by his father because he looks ill. On the way home he collapses:

I looked up, and beheld the same messenger standing over my head, surrounded by light as before. He then again re-

---

[4] Although Mormon historian Quinn ascribes this triplicity to necromantic custom in the magic world view (33), the treble visitation of Joseph's surgeons to his leg might easily have been the more significant factor.

> lated unto me all that he had related to me the previous
> night, and commanded me to go to my father and tell him of
> the vision. . . .
>
> I obeyed; I returned to my father in the field, and re-
> hearsed the whole matter to him. He replied to me that it was
> of God, and told me to go and do as commanded by the mes-
> senger. I left the field, and went to the place where the mes-
> senger had told me the plates were deposited; and owing to
> the distinctness of the vision which I had had concerning it,
> I knew the place the instant that I arrived there. (34)

This final afterthought, in which Joseph's father enters the story to lend his essential imprimatur, is the link between the First Vision and the Second. In each case there are two authority figures, not one, and in each case the father's role is to pronounce the legitimacy of the messenger, who, in turn, passes the torch of responsibility to Joseph. The Book of Ether's message repeats.

It is more than a little interesting that in Joseph's first publication of this vision, as well as in the description of this vision in his mother's biography, the name Nephi rather than Moroni was used to describe the messenger. In later versions the earlier name was declared to be erroneous. The "error," however, may carry much more meaning than its subsequent correction, especially in the context of a Freudian slip. Since the transfer of responsibility to Joseph at this critical moment for the beginning of his work of grandeur is again the theme of the Book of Ether, the evidence would suggest that the personage in the vision is again a representation of Alvin. Comment was made on p. 79 on Joseph's playing on the letters of his own name (JOS and JOE in the page of "reformed Egyptian" characters given to Martin Harris). The central three letters of Nephi's name (eph) are in fact the final three letters of Joseph's name, and the two that bracket it are the final two of Alvin's, with the statistical likelihood of this having occurred randomly being about one in a hundred million. How better to symbolize the passing of the torch than with a hybrid name? Joseph would become the firstborn by melding himself with Alvin in the creation of Nephi, the protagonist of his fantasy—the paragon that Joseph imagined himself to have become in Alvin's firstborn image. The grieving did not stop.

Alvin's death and the horrid exhumation that followed it did indeed represent a second emotional trauma for Joseph, but it was of a special kind: a bereavement trauma. As Terr notes in her classic work on childhood trauma (35), bereavement is especially difficult for youngsters when accompanied by the utter helplessness of the traumatic condition. Children tend to have longstanding difficulties with deaths of those close to them because they process losses more slowly than do adults. They must go through the same phases of mourning: denial, protest, despair with repetitious reworkings of the relationship, and final resolution or detachment. But whereas adults usually complete the process in a year or so, children may spend years in just one phase in their inability to say a permanent good-bye. Although Joseph was hardly a child at seventeen, his personality was doubtless hobbled in specific ways by his earlier trauma, and the record suggests that he did not grieve for Alvin hastily.

Bereavement trauma, says Terr, produces some of the most bizarre behavior of all—often resulting in misdiagnosis as schizophrenia. The potent bereavement/trauma combination frequently induces paranormal experiences and hallucinations as vivid reenactments and fantasies. Children in this state even see ghosts of dead family members.[5] "If you scare a child badly enough," Terr points out, "he will be traumatized—plain and simple. But if you combine the trauma with a death or a new disability, then you will see depression, paranormal thinking, and/or character change—count on it" (37).

Both the First and Second Visions have content that strongly suggests Alvin's presence in just such a hallucination. In the First Vision is seen the father-brother duality with the underlying theme of torch-passing as in the Book of Ether. The Second Vision, carrying the identical theme, is prologue to the anniversary ritual over Alvin's exhumation. That both are described in the exquisite and minute visual detail typical of the

---

[5] Terr's study of the 1986 *Challenger* disaster demonstrated, for example, that a remarkable 41% of high school students who had viewed the actual explosion as it happened had some form of subsequent paranormal experience such as a hallucination related to the event (36).

posttraumatic trance gives special significance to Terr's observation:

> Saintly visions, as recorded by the Church, include the precision of detail and the vivid colorations that you also "see" in the visual experiences of traumatized kids. Yes, perhaps the saints *were* traumatized—at least some of them. (38)

Theophanies, perhaps. Fratroscopies, more likely.

In a seamless pattern another such vision occurs as Joseph nears completion of *The Book of Mormon*. While praying in the woods with Oliver Cowdery on May 15, 1829, he receives directions from "a messenger from heaven" that they baptize each other and enter the "Aaronic" priesthood. Joseph's narrative continues: "The messenger who visited us on this occasion, and conferred this Priesthood upon us, said that his name was John, the same that is called John the Baptist in the New Testament" (39). Again, it is not God the Father in the theophany but a "messenger" who passes the torch to Joseph—a repetition of the theme of the story of the brother of Jared. This detail supports the identification of Alvin with John the Baptist in Joseph's mind, presaging the coming of one much greater, namely himself. As one senses the message of the torch being passed, there is an implicit message that Joseph saw that it was somehow Alvin's prerogative, and his alone, to confer this station upon his "chosen successor," since the Aaronic priesthood, according to Joseph's prophecy, was to remain a strictly familial affiliation, with eligibility determined solely by virtue of being "a literal descendent of Aaron."

It is further important to remember the timing of Joseph's founding of the church, as was noted in the same context on p. 142 in connection with the translation of the plates. Because Alvin had died at the age of twenty-five, Joseph seems to have identified this age as the critical one in his own life for taking up Alvin's fallen mantle. As is common in anniversary reactions, the onset of unusual behavior patterns frequently coincides with the age when a parent or other closely identified person previously underwent a major life event, usually of a tragic nature (40, 41). If Joseph was to complete his preparations and build the church that he associated with Alvin, it had to be accomplished about 1830, when he was in his twenty-fifth year of age. He maintained his timetable well.

Additional clues to Joseph's feelings toward Alvin are seen in an 1836 "vision" in Kirtland, Ohio, which Joseph described as follows:

> The heavens were opened upon us, and I beheld the celestial kingdom of God, and the glory thereof . . . also the blazing throne of God, whereon was seated the Father and the Son. I saw the beautiful streets of that kingdom, which had the appearance of being paved with gold. I saw Fathers Adam and Abraham, and my father and mother, my brother, Alvin, that has long since slept, and marvelled how it was that he had obtained an inheritance in that kingdom, seeing that he had departed this life before the Lord had set His hand to gather Israel the second time, and had not been baptized for the remission of sins. (42)

Clearly, Alvin is placed in distinguished patriarchal company in this passage alongside "Fathers Adam and Abraham" and Joseph's own parents. This further supports the view that Alvin occupied an auxiliary paternal role in Joseph's mind.

There is also a suggestion in this passage that Joseph is more than a little troubled over the issue of Alvin's death. Despite the religious brush with which this uneasiness is painted, one can glimpse a specter of Alvin having been deprived of something and that Joseph was in some way responsible. Yet, despite Joseph's failure to have been able to include Alvin in the fellowship of those whom he had baptized into celestial glory, Joseph's fantasy on this occasion puts Alvin there in the most exalted company anyway. It is this fantasy of saving Alvin—of somehow making up for some heartfelt shortcoming of the past—that dominates the passage and that makes more understandable the "revelation" that follows immediately after the above passage: "All who have died without a knowledge of this Gospel, who would have received it if they had been permitted to tarry, shall be heirs of the celestial kingdom of God" (43).

The meaning of the juxtaposition of this revelation with Joseph's troubled fantasy concerning Alvin's salvation is clear. Joseph's perceived need to "do right" by Alvin seems greater than the actual facts of an unexpected family death of years ago would warrant. One again suspects that guilt is playing no small role in Joseph's unresolved grief over his older brother's death. The fantasy on this occasion expresses the wish for a reunion with Alvin so that Joseph could "make up" to him for having usurped his firstborn role. Joseph's wish is therefore grandly expanded into a divine pronouncement that changes all of the previous rules about the prerequisites for eschatological reward. The fantasy apparently reassures Joseph that his wish will be fulfilled.

But even this action on Alvin's behalf appears to have been insufficient to resolve Joseph's lingering grief over the troubling circumstances of his brother's death. The revelation and its accompanying fantasy of Alvin in celestial glory, though seemingly ample in their content to have made up for any prior shortcoming, apparently were still too vague. A more direct and personal intercession would be needed.

Joseph had for some time been fascinated with notions of heaven and hell. He had posed a schema wherein all departed souls resided in a kind of holding place until the Day of Judgment. One could make a kind of shortcut to avoid this purgatory-like phase of the afterlife only by having been baptized into Joseph's church. It was this criterion, unmet by Alvin, that seemed to trouble Joseph—especially because of some personal responsibility that the prophet evidently felt for this state of affairs. After all, Joseph held full responsibility through his revelations for having established the new order, and he could see that he had left out a provision for Alvin's salvation.

For the final absolution, Alvin would need somehow to be formally baptized. But short of a second hideous exhumation, how could this be accomplished? In the course of his troubled ruminations over his mixed feelings toward Alvin, Joseph would devise a way—one that was imaginative and ingenious. He would stand in for the dead brother with whom he identified and would be baptized on his behalf, receiving absolution for his lingering guilt in the process. He could "make it right" by an act of submission, identification, and penance. Once again, Joseph's inner conflicts seem to have sought resolution in an overt act of public religious ritual.

"Baptism for the dead" became a unique sacrament of Mormonism. Joseph wrote of the new practice in a letter to his missionaries in England in the fall of 1840:

> The Saints have the privilege of being baptized for those of their relatives who are dead, whom they believe would have embraced the Gospel, if they had been privileged with hearing it, and who have received the Gospel in the spirit, through the instrumentality of those who have been commissioned to preach to them while in prison. (44)

And these baptisms for the dead could not properly be performed in just any convenient river. Joseph's new revelation on the subject specified the following:

> For a baptismal font there is not upon the earth, that they, my saints, may be baptized for those who are dead. For this ordinance belongeth to my house . . . For it is ordained that in Zion, and in her Stakes, and in Jerusalem, those places which I have appointed for refuge, shall be the places for your baptisms for your dead. (45)

Only a temple of supreme grandeur would be fitting for such an important endeavor. Whatever inner force drove Joseph to pay such tribute to Alvin, it was indeed a powerful one.

It is worth noting that although the early Mormon community was a closely knit but heterogeneous fellowship of believers, Joseph restricted the practice of baptism for the dead only to "relatives," as described in his letter to England. With Joseph's admitted admiration for American patriots who had gone on before, as well as for writers whose works he admired for various reasons, Joseph could easily have extended the sacrament to include "great persons" as well as "friends." The fact that he chose not to do so lends further support to the concept that baptism for the dead was created for a very special relative—almost certainly the one for whom the Book of Ether was written.

But it is the timing of the introduction of this sacrament that is its most interesting feature. Unlike the sacrament of celestial marriage, whose roots were sunk into the earliest days of the movement, baptism for the dead seems to have appeared virtually de novo in the fall of 1840. Aside from an occasional cryptic reference to the fact that "the hearts of the children shall turn to their fathers," there seem to be no premonitory sermons or writings by Joseph on the subject that are apparent in the public record, and the earlier references to the theological problem of souls who died without having been baptized into Mormonism (such as in his 1836 Kirtland vision and revelation) contradict the need for such a sacrament by making salvation automatic if it could be judged that any such souls "would have received" the new Gospel if they had been alive.

The missing piece in the chronology may be the almost exact correspondence between the introduction of baptism for the dead and the death of Joseph's father on September 14, 1840. Joseph Smith, Sr. had been in failing health during the spring and summer of 1840. By late summer it was clear that he was on his deathbed. On August 10, 1840, one month before his moribund father would die, Joseph first spoke in public about his new sacrament. Not surprisingly, the occasion he chose was a funeral sermon, as the matter of death was undoubtedly much on his mind at this time (46). Three weeks after his father's death, Joseph took the floor at a meeting of the General Conference of the church and "delivered a discourse on the subject of baptism for the dead, which was listened to with considerable interest, by the vast multitude assembled" (47). The fact that this discourse was sandwiched between discussions of the Nauvoo city plat and the need for a city charter would suggest that the prophet was a bit preoccupied at the time by this troubling issue. The following day an article by the prophet on the Priesthood was read to the conference. The article contained two long digressions into matters of resurrection of the dead and communications with the dead. Five days later, on October 10, he wrote the letter to the British missionaries from which a passage was quoted above. The formal revelation on the subject followed on January 19, 1841, and subsequent writings by Joseph appeared on the subject into the fall of 1842.

In September of 1842, significantly the month of both the second anniversary of his father's death and the eighteenth anniversary of Alvin's exhumation, Joseph wrote to his parishioners: "I now resume the subject of baptism for the dead, as that subject seems to occupy my mind, and press itself upon my feelings the strongest . . ." The lengthy letter about his sacrament continued:

> Herein is glory, and honor, and immortality, and eternal life: The ordinance of baptism by water, to be immersed therein in order to answer to the likeness of the dead, that one principle might accord with the other. To be immersed in the water and come forth out of the water is in the likeness of the resurrection of the dead, in coming forth out of their graves . . . Consequently, the baptismal font was instituted as a simile of the grave, and was commanded to be in a place underneath where the living are wont to assemble, to show forth the living and the dead, and that all things may have their likeness, and that they may accord one with another . . .
>
> For we without them cannot be made perfect; neither can they without us be made perfect. (48)

The sorrow, unresolved grief, and longing for the protective presence of the departed lingered for Joseph as he tried to expunge these feelings through repetitive ritual. The pointed reference to "coming forth out of their graves" and the design of the baptismal font to resemble a grave seem as dissociated repetitions of the exhumation of Alvin, the event so troubling to Joseph. And again, one senses that some kind of unfulfilled obligation toward a dead relative was ever-present. The final sentence of the above passage, in particular, seems to represent an acknowledgment of Alvin's sacrifice on Joseph's behalf as well as Joseph's need to repay his own guilty debt to Alvin. Joseph owed Alvin as Alvin owed Joseph.

The connection between Alvin and the sacrament of baptism for the dead has not, in fact, been obscure in the historical record. Joseph's mother, in her narrative of the deathbed conversation between the prophet and his father, relates that "Joseph came in and told his father . . . that it was then the privilege of the Saints to be baptized for the dead. [This] Mr. Smith was delighted to hear, and requested, that Joseph should be baptized for Alvin immediately" (49). Joseph, Sr., too, evidently still ached over the loss of his firstborn.

It would be easy from this exchange and from the known chronology to conclude that Joseph had conceived this sacrament merely to please his father on his deathbed. Knowing of his father's lingering grief over Alvin's death, Joseph surely understood what comfort this message would bring to the dying man. It is therefore tempting to conclude that the sacrament, having taken form over the years in Joseph's thoughts, was brought forward at this moment in the story for this intimate family purpose.

But was the timing really so rational? Perhaps not. Joseph may in fact have been dealing with a nonrational motive in establishing baptism for the dead when he did. The new ritual may instead have been propelled out of the depths of his troubled psyche by the appearance of his father on his deathbed, the specter reawakening the bitter memory of Alvin's death and the dissociated image of Alvin's half-decomposed corpse. Did the impending death of his father, impacting so cruelly upon Joseph by its occurrence in mid-September, bring back the pain and guilt of the loss of his brother nearly two decades before? That the season of mid-September had long elicited grief-stricken rituals toward Alvin on Joseph's part may point toward the solution to the puzzle over the timing. That the anniversary even continued to drive him thereafter is suggested by the fact that it was in September of 1842, two years later, that, as noted above, Joseph wrote of baptism of the dead, "as that subject seems to occupy my mind, and press itself upon my feelings the strongest."

Psychiatrist Erich Lindemann noted that the "most striking and most frequent" feature of normal and distorted grief responses among relatives of those who have died suddenly is "*delay* or *postponement*" (50). He concludes:

> That this delay may involve years became obvious first by the fact that patients in acute bereavement about a recent death may soon upon exploration be found preoccupied with grief about a person who died many years ago. In this manner a woman of 38, whose mother had died recently and

who had responded to the mother's death with a surprisingly severe reaction, was found to be but mildly concerned with her mother's death but deeply engrossed with unhappy and perplexing fantasies concerning the death of her brother, who died twenty years ago under dramatic circumstances from metastasizing carcinoma after amputation of his arm had been postponed too long. The discovery that a former unresolved grief reaction may be precipitated in the course of the discussion of another recent event was soon demonstrated in psychiatric interviews by patients who showed all the traits of a true grief reaction when the topic of a former loss arose. (51)

It is this sort of reaction that seems the more likely explanation for the sudden appearance of this sacrament around the time of Joseph Smith, Sr.'s death. Certainly the elder Smith did not require the posthumous sacrament himself, since he had been baptized a decade before in upstate New York. As with the patient Lindemann describes, Joseph, Jr.'s reaction and the ritual it spawned seem to be centered more on the dramatic earlier death of his older brother and its aftermath than on that of his parent. It is unlikely that Joseph was sufficiently prospective in his theological planning to have designed this new sacrament merely as a balm for family members on the occasion of the paternal deathbed watch.

The symbolic importance of the death of Joseph's father must not be discounted in its own right, however. Freud has pointed out that the death of the father is often the most important event in a man's life (52). Because this is the moment when he "succeeds," or replaces, his father, the event may rekindle the powerful emotions of childhood toward the father. Several writers, including Freud, have noted, for example, that *Hamlet* was written immediately after the death of Shakespeare's own father. Psychoanalyst Ernest Jones emphasized the feeling of death throughout this play and the fact that the play deals with the death of both a father and a father-substitute; he also noted that the play marked the author's career turning point from comedy to tragedy (53). There is thus a strong suggestion that the play is a statement of Shakespeare's own unresolved oedipal conflict, presumably in this case a literary expression of those reawakened childhood feelings associated with the death of his own father.[6]

It is likely that these matters had significance for Joseph and his own creative expressivity as well, at least to the extent that Alvin had earlier served as an auxiliary father. The issue of the "murder" of Alvin, or at least of having had to deal with the guilt of usurping his "first-born" position, perhaps represented a disturbing oedipal theme that was stirred up at the death of Joseph's father. In addition, reawakening of the buried oedipal feelings surrounding his earlier surgical tragedy should have surrounded his father's demise. The two deaths, viewed together, were so abhorrent that only the plaint of the new ritual could defend against the guilt and pain. It was at his father's deathbed, as much as with *The Book of Mormon,* that his childhood surgical trauma confronted his teenage tragedy. Killing the father was a different issue for Joseph than killing a brother. One he had forever dreaded as the forbidden act. The other he seems to have experienced in all its awful pain and was forever haunted by it. And as at other such defining moments in Joseph's troubled life, a unique ritual would memorialize it.

Joseph Smith, Jr. would grieve in many ways for Alvin. Was there something specific in the family's reaction to the tragic event of 1823 that had prevented a healthy resolution of young Joseph's bereavement at the time? Was there a perceived accusation of blame toward Joseph, Jr. in some casual comment of the parents during their own difficult time? Were the parents, through insensitivity or anger at the doctor or minister, unable to assist their remaining children through their own difficult grieving? Was the rapid transfer of the parents' mantle of expectation from firstborn Alvin onto their middle child too great a burden for him to bear alongside his own confused grief and guilt over Alvin's loss? The answers will never be known.

One thing is clear, however. Joseph's longing for Alvin has resulted in a legacy of inestimable value to genealogists. For what he

---

[6] Hamlet's inability to avenge his father's death in Jones's view is seen as an expression of the fact that he saw himself as no less guilty than the murderer himself.

created in the ritualistic expression of his delayed bereavement required not only that his followers baptize their dead relatives but that they first find out who those relatives were. Stored securely inside Granite Mountain in Utah's majestic Wasatch Range are microfilm rolls bearing nearly two billion names, intertwining Latter-day Saints into vastly extended families of humankind through the ages—a permanent and lasting monument to Joseph's grief.

Notes

1. Levy D: "Psychic Trauma of Operations in Children." *American Journal of Diseases of Children* 69:7–25, 1945.
2. Brodie F: *No Man Knows My History: The Life of Joseph Smith, the Mormon Prophet,* 2nd Edition. New York, Alfred A. Knopf, 1989, pp. 414–416.
3. Bettelheim B: *The Uses of Enchantment: The Meaning and Importance of Fairy Tales.* New York, Vintage Books, 1975, pp. 102–111.
4. Smith J: *The Book of the Law of the Lord,* entry of 23 August 1842. Salt Lake City, LDS Church Archives (First Presidency's Vault), pp. 179–180. See also Vogel D (ed): *Early Mormon Documents,* Vol. 1. Salt Lake City, Signature Books, 1996, p. 175.
5. Quinn M: *Early Mormonism and the Magic World View.* Salt Lake City, Signature Books, 1987, p. 135.
6. Cain AC, Cain BS: "On Replacing a Child." *Journal of the American Academy of Child Psychiatry* 3:443–456, 1964.
7. Cain AC, Fast I, Erickson ME: "Children's Disturbed Reactions to the Death of a Sibling." *American Journal of Orthopsychiatry* 34:741–752, 1964.
8. Ibid., p. 743.
9. Ibid., pp. 744–745.
10. Record of the trial of Joseph Smith for disorderly conduct, Bainbridge, NY, March 20, 1826. Published in the *New Schaff–Herzog Encyclopedia of Religious Knowledge,* Vol. 2. New York, 1883, p. 1576. Cited in Brodie F: *No Man Knows My History,* 2nd Edition, pp. 428–429.

11. Terr L: *Unchained Memories: True Stories of Traumatic Memories, Lost and Found.* New York, Basic Books, 1994, p. 162.

12. Inman WS: "Clinical Observations on Morbid Periodicity." *British Journal of Medical Psychology* 21:254–262, 1948.

13. Hilgard JR, Newman MF: "Anniversaries in Mental Illness," in *Theory and Practice of Family Psychiatry.* Edited by Howells JG. Edinburgh, Oliver & Boyd, 1968, pp. 635–646.

14. Smith W: *William Smith on Mormonism.* Lamoni, IA, Herald Steam Book & Job Office, 1896, pp. 5–19. Cited in Vogel D (ed): *Early Mormon Documents,* Vol. 1, p. 496.

15. Butterworth CE: "The Old Soldier's Testimony." Sermon preached by Bro. William B. Smith, in the Saints' Chapel, Detroit, IA, June 8, 1884. *Saints' Herald* 31:643–644, 1884. Cited in Vogel D (ed): *Early Mormon Documents,* Vol. 1, pp. 504–505.

16. Vogel D (ed): *Early Mormon Documents,* Vol. 1, pp. 325 (n. 132), 327 (n. 135).

17. Salisbury KS: "Dear Sisters." *Saints' Herald* 33:260, 1886. Cited in Vogel D (ed): *Early Mormon Documents,* Vol. 1, p. 521.

18. Chase W: "Affidavit," in Howe ED: *Mormonism Unvailed.* Painesville, OH, 1834, pp. 240–248.

19. Quinn M: *Early Mormonism and the Magic World View,* p. 127.

20. See Jessee DC: "Joseph Knight's Recollection of Early Mormon History." *BYU Studies* 17:29–39, 1976.

21. See Persuitte D: *Joseph Smith and the Origins of The Book of Mormon.* Jefferson, NC, McFarland & Company, 1985, pp. 69–71.

22. Harris H: "Affidavit," in Howe ED: *Mormonism Unvailed,* pp. 251–252.

23. Brodie F: *No Man Knows My History,* 2nd Edition, p. 410.

24. Vogel D (ed): *Early Mormon Documents,* Vol. 1, p. 55.

25. See Howe ED: *Mormonism Unvailed,* p. 269.

26. Quoted in Howe ED: *Mormonism Unvailed,* p. 267.

27. Chase W: "Affidavit," in Howe ED: *Mormonism Unvailed,* pp. 246–247.

28. Laws of New York, Forty-Second Session, Chapter CCXVII, 1819, p. 279 [courtesy of Cultural Education Center, New York State Historical Society].
29. Brodie F: *No Man Knows My History*, p. 25.
30. Smith J: *Manuscript History of the Church*, Book A-1. Salt Lake City, LDS Church Archives, 1838, p. 3. Quoted in Vogel D (ed): *Early Mormon Documents*, Vol. 1, pp. 60–61.
31. Smith J: *Manuscript History of the Church*, Book A-1, p. 5. Quoted in Vogel D (ed): *Early Mormon Documents*, Vol. 1, pp. 63–64.
32. Smith J: *Manuscript History of the Church*, Book A-1, p. 6. Quoted in Vogel D (ed): *Early Mormon Documents*, Vol. 1, p. 65.
33. Quinn M: *Early Mormonism and the Magic World View*, pp. 115–116.
34. Smith J: *Manuscript History of the Church*, Book A-1, p. 7. Quoted in Vogel D (ed): *Early Mormon Documents*, Vol. 1, p. 6.
35. Terr L: *Too Scared to Cry: Psychic Trauma in Childhood.* New York, Harper & Row, 1990, pp. 97–108.
36. Terr L: *Unchained Memories*, p. 200.
37. Terr L: *Too Scared to Cry*, p. 107.
38. Ibid., p. 134.
39. Smith J: *Manuscript History of the Church*, Book A-1, p. 18. Quoted in Vogel D (ed): *Early Mormon Documents*, Vol. 1, p. 75.
40. Hilgard JR, Newman MF: "Anniversaries in Mental Illness," in *Theory and Practice of Family Psychiatry.* Edited by Howells JG. Edinburgh, Oliver & Boyd, 1968, pp. 635–646.
41. Hilgard JR: "Anniversary Reactions in Parents Precipitated by Children." *Psychiatry* 16:73–80, 1953.
42. Smith J: *History of the Church of Jesus Christ of Latter-day Saints*, Vol. II. Annotated by Roberts BH. Salt Lake City, Deseret Book Company, 1927, p. 380.
43. Smith J: *History of the Church of Jesus Christ of Latter-day Saints*, Vol. II, p. 380.

44. Smith J: *History of the Church of Jesus Christ of Latter-day Saints,* Vol. IV. Annotated by Roberts BH. Salt Lake City, Deseret Book Company, 1927, p. 231.

45. *Doctrine and Covenants,* Section 124, vv. 29–30, 36. Salt Lake City, Deseret News Company, 1880, pp. 432–433.

46. Smith J: *History of the Church of Jesus Christ of Latter-day Saints,* Vol. IV, p. 179.

47. Ibid., p. 206.

48. *Doctrine and Covenants,* Section 128, vv. 12–13, 18, pp. 454–456.

49. Smith LM: *Biographical Sketches of Joseph Smith the Prophet and His Progenitors for Many Generations.* Liverpool, S. W. Richards, 1853 [reprinted New York, Arno Press, 1969], pp. 265–266.

50. Lindemann E: "Symptomatology and Management of Acute Grief." *American Journal of Psychiatry* 101:141–148, 1944; see p. 144.

51. Ibid., p. 144.

52. Freud S: *The Interpretation of Dreams* (1900). Translated by Brill AA. New York, Macmillan Co., 1913, pp. 224–225.

53. Jones E: *Hamlet and Oedipus.* Garden City, NY, Doubleday, 1955, pp. 128–130.1

Chapter Seven

The Arrows of Eros

A s publication of *The Book of Mormon* drew near, Joseph arranged for some of those who believed in his "gift" to provide public corroboration of his powers. In a June 1829 prophecy delivered to Oliver Cowdery, Martin Harris, and friend David Whitmer, Joseph proclaimed:

> Behold, I say unto you, that you must rely upon my word, which if you do with full purpose of heart, you shall have a view of the plates, and also the breastplate, the sword of Laban, the Urim and Thummim, which were given to the brother of Jared upon the mount, when he talked with the Lord face to face, and the miraculous directors which were given to Lehi while in the wilderness, on the borders of the Red Sea. (1)

Something new has been introduced in this passage. Heretofore, in his own description of events, Joseph had alleged finding only the gold

plates, at least one pair of magic stones, and the breastplate in the
box at Hill Cumorah, as cited in Chapter 4. His mother, in her recollection (2), however, and Joseph Knight, in his (3), both refer to
Joseph, Jr.'s accounts to them of his setting aside the plates in
search of "something else" of great value in the box. Oliver Cowdery recalled Joseph's perusal of the contents of the box for something that "would still add to his store of wealth" (4).

A significant unanswered question remained in Chapter 4
concerning the identity of this unfound object in the box at Hill
Cumorah—the object of greater worth than the engraved record
of the ancients and the magic translator-stones and the object toward which Joseph's greed was so great that his avarice caused
forfeiture of the right to acquire the plates. That object of inestimable worth—the sword of Laban—is now placed by Joseph into
his contemporary world for the first time. The central talisman of
The Book of Mormon, the dissociated image of Nathan Smith's
fearsome amputation knife, was for Joseph the ultimate power
symbol. He would introduce the sword of Laban into the opening
pages of *The Book of Mormon,* carry it through the chapters of the
book to a climactic burial, resurrect it through the sexual symbolism of a treasure search, and, finally, brandish it triumphantly before witnesses. And nine years later, one of Joseph's armed band
of defenders in Missouri would write to a fellow Mormon in a letter, "Come to Zion and fight for the religion of Jesus. Many a hoary
head is engaged here, the Prophet goes out to the battle as in days
of old. He has the sword that Nephi took from Laban. Is not this
marvellous?" (5). By possessing this object himself in fantasy, Joseph gained the omnipotence and invincibility that it symbolized.
Like a boy dreaming of his surgery, he now held the horrible scalpel and all the awesome power that had once confronted him.

Regardless of the mechanism by which the witnessing took
place (for the historical record is muddied with disparate recollections), Joseph was able to obtain the signatures of eleven men
to two separate statements supporting his claim to the ancient
treasures. The statements were published on the final two pages
of *The Book of Mormon.* That Joseph himself wrote the statements is strongly suggested by his characteristic phrasing, the use
of the imagery of blood on garments, and the fact that the text

agreed completely with his own accounts rather than those given later by at least one of the signatories. The first statement describes a mystical event, the second a sort of exhibition.

But publishing *The Book of Mormon* was one thing; distributing it would be quite another. By making the book more means than end, Joseph may have used the book as a marketing tool to sell himself and not vice versa. As the text of *The Book of Mormon* presupposed a new religious movement, Joseph founded his church eleven days following publication, proclaiming himself a "Seer, a Translator, a Prophet, an Apostle of Jesus Christ, and Elder of the Church through the will of God the Father, and the grace of your Lord Jesus Christ" (6).

The tiny cult of Smith family members and believing friends stirred angry passions among skeptical neighbors and townsfolk, who were only too familiar with the necromantic activities of *The Book of Mormon*'s author. The first weeks and months of the tiny new church were precarious for the life and limb of the founders, even as abundant door-to-door sales and distribution of the book swelled the membership among those in towns and villages where Joseph's tainted reputation was not so appreciated. But soon the struggling group would be given a quantum boost in strength when the charismatic Campbellite preacher Sidney Rigdon professed his belief in the divinity of *The Book of Mormon* and brought his own Ohio followers into the fold. Joseph left New York State for Ohio in January 1831, together with his devoted band of sixty disciples, in the first westward leg of one of the most unusual institutional odysseys in the history of the United States.

Since this phase of frontier history has been thoroughly chronicled by historians, it is not necessary here to detail the eventful economic and social interactions of this burgeoning society other than to allude to the brief narrative provided in Chapter 1. Suffice it to say that Joseph Smith, Jr. maintained, by dint of his personal resourcefulness and growing charisma, firm control of the dynamic organization despite recurring crises from within and without. Borrowing concepts of communal property sharing from his Campbellite associates, Joseph established islands of socialistic theocracy on the frontier, with himself as both spiritual and fiduciary leader, and with nearly every faithful adult male appointed to some form of priesthood office. Always financially undercapitalized, the rapidly growing organization coaxed away the personal assets of new converts in futile efforts to catch its inaccessible tail of collective indebtedness. From Kirtland, Ohio, to western Missouri and back to the Mississippi River at Nauvoo, Illinois, the group fled from creditors, political enemies, and social and religious detractors, all the while swelling in numbers and in fealty to its undaunted prophet.

But Joseph's inner turmoil would be no less with him in triumph than in poverty. The torment in his mind continued to vent itself in ways that can be glimpsed at many notable intervals throughout the narrative. Although many are of no more than passing consequence, some of these nuances in behavior appear to have become entombed in lasting effigy within the structure, ritual, and tradition of the church he founded.

One such important behavioral pattern may be introduced with an event known to nearly all Latter-day Saints. In March of 1832, Joseph and Emma were living near Kirtland, Ohio, with the Johnson family, one of whose members Joseph had apparently healed of a lame arm. Emma had recently lost both of a set of twins in childbirth for the second successive natal tragedy the couple had had to bear. Shortly thereafter, when another set of twins was born in Kirtland to a mother who had died in the course of delivery, the infants were given to Joseph and Emma to raise. With both twins shortly contracting measles, Joseph was conducting a post-midnight vigil with the more ill of the two when a drunken mob smashed into the Johnson home, bent on tarring and feathering the Mormon prophet.

One might well imagine that Joseph experienced more than a little sense of déjà vu on this occasion. Occupying the bedside of a suffering small boy should by itself have aroused some uncomfortable lingering memories. The unwelcome and unanticipated entry of an assault force of men at this moment must have evoked as much sheer terror as he had experienced during the original awful events of nineteen years before. Although an eyewitness account placed the number of attackers at "forty or fifty" (7), it is significant that Joseph, in his own recollection, described a more familiar number: "I found myself going out of the door, in the hands of about a dozen men" (8), the same number burned into his mind from the earlier assault and indeed the number central to much of his life's ritual. Had there been two hundred on this occasion, one suspects he would still have imagined there were "about a dozen men." (A famous mural in Salt Lake City shows the twelve assailants of Joseph's own account.)

What is known of Joseph's behavior on this occasion further suggests that the event represented something more than its face value to the prophet. One William Waste, widely regarded as "the strongest man on the Western Reserve," had boasted he could take Joseph out of the Johnson house by himself. Mormon accounts of the episode proudly describe Joseph's flattening of Waste with one kick in terms that suggest a tribute to the prophet's personal strength and virility (9, 10). Luke Johnson quotes Waste as saying later that Joseph was "the most powerful man he ever had hold of in his life" (11). Although such a statement is undoubtedly true, the strength displayed on that occasion must not be regarded as Joseph's customary power but rather as resulting from the severest kind of adrenaline rush. Waste and his comrades had found themselves facing a thrice-traumatized seven-year-old fending off a fourth mortal assault on his manhood. Joseph screamed for mercy as he was stretched out on a large board and stripped of his clothes. Nitric acid was forced into his mouth, and a tooth was chipped. He was scratched, beaten, taunted, and tarred and feathered.

But these insults, painful and humiliating though they were, paled before the real threat. It seems that a physician was part of the mob. A Dr. Dennison had been persuaded to join the assault and to bring along his set of surgical instruments to perform the unthinkable act. The oaths shouted at Joseph while he was restrained on the board were prelude to the literal emasculation that was planned as the climax to the event. He saw the doctor approach with his surgical instruments in what must have been the single most terrifying moment of his adult life. On encountering the prostrate man, however, Dr. Dennison was unable or unwilling to proceed and withdrew, leaving Joseph's manhood physically intact. The prophet was merely beaten unconscious and deserted on the cold March ground (12, 13, 14).

Joseph's own description of his experience, as related through a friend, is most revealing: ". . . his [Joseph's] spirit seemed to leave his body, and during the period of insensibility he consciously stood over his own body, feeling no pain, but seeing and hearing all that transpired" (15). This statement is a textbook description of dissociation. Joseph retreats wholly into the split-off world of his mind, able to induce a self-hypnotic trance that separates him completely from the pain of reality. In Terr's words, "Dissociation is a mechanism that enables a person to quit a place where bad thoughts or events are happening" (16). Such experiences are seen very frequently as learned responses among victims of *repetitive* childhood trauma as protective reactions. Such individuals, Terr states, "tend to separate themselves from these attacks as they happen, creating spontaneous self-hypnosis and massive denial" (17).

The parallels for Joseph between this adult event and the childhood trauma he experienced do not end with his dissociative self-hypnosis and the physical similarities of the two assaults. It seems that the mob's motive for selecting emasculation as the proper punishment had little to do with Joseph's religious views. Eli Johnson, an older brother in the host family, appears to have arranged for the surgical dismemberment because of his anger over Joseph's intimacies with his sixteen-year-old sister, Nancy Marinda Johnson. It is likely that Eli and his friends conveyed this fact to Joseph in the clearest of terms in the moments before Dr. Dennison's arrival. Joseph's screams for mercy must therefore be seen in the context in which he uttered them: not as the plaint of an innocent victim of religious persecution, but as the guilt-laden pleas of one who had engaged in forbidden sexuality and had been discovered—precisely the predicament in fantasy under which he had faced the assault nearly two decades before. This time, Eli Johnson played the jealous, rivalrous father role, and Dr. Dennison stood in for the evil paternal accomplice, Dr. Nathan Smith; the rest of the mob played medical students—the "Council of Surgeons."

On emerging from unconsciousness, Joseph stumbled home to spend the rest of the night undergoing removal of the tar by his wife and her friends. As he was scheduled to preach the next

morning, many of his assailants waited gleefully in the congregation. Joseph reportedly arrived on schedule and delivered a dignified sermon to the astonishment of those who had anticipated
a different kind of spectacle. It is said that this so impressed a sizable number on this occasion that many were inspired to join
ranks with this remarkable man. Knowing, however, of the childhood precursor to this particular event, one might wonder if the
sermon wasn't more likely a benumbed, shame-inspired act of
contrite redemption than a manifestation of the serene strength
of an innocent martyr.

The point was emphasized in Chapter 3 that repetition of
a stressful stimulus is a powerful force in strengthening the development of abnormal mind functions. It is therefore likely that this
violent event, so closely paralleling the circumstances of the
nightmarish incident of Joseph's childhood, strongly reinforced
the fantasies and dissociative forces still actively churning just
outside of conscious memory from that already thrice-repeated
event of fantasied dismemberment. Eroticism and the threat of
violence would be yet more tightly fused in Joseph's mind.

Nancy Marinda Johnson had indeed been an object of Joseph's
passion. So, with little doubt, had others before her, and so would
there be many, many more. The pattern of expression of this passion, so consistent, repetitive, and almost ritualistic from woman
to woman, was sufficiently bizarre in the aggregate that it merits
closest scrutiny. To understand the origin of this aberrant behavior would be to understand a root cause of much of the Mormon
conflict on the American frontier.

Indeed, if there is one feature of Mormon history that is popu-
larly recognized as most distinctive, it is undoubtedly the practice
of polygamy. The responsibility for the conception and introduction of this practice belongs squarely with Joseph Smith, Jr. The
historical record on this point is clear and unambiguous. But to
dismiss Joseph's sexual behavior as mere rakish promiscuity, as
some Mormon detractors have done, is to miss the central feature
of a complex structure of ego defenses built to deal with some
very troublesome conflicts.

The record of Joseph's adolescent and early adult years is understandably scanty concerning his private sexual behavior.

There is the general affidavit signed by 51 residents of Palmyra, New York, that "Joseph Smith Senior, and his son Joseph, were in particular, considered entirely destitute of *moral character, and addicted to vicious habits . . .*," and Joseph Capron swore that members of the Smith family were "addicted to vice and the grossest immoralities" (18).[1] Clark Braden reported that

> Dr. McIntyre, family physician of the Smith's in Manchester, N. Y., declares that the house of Joseph Smith, Sr., was a perfect brothel. Ezra Pierce, Samantha Payne and other schoolmates and associates of the Smith's, testify that Smith was lewd, and so were the family and the entire money hunting gang, and that the digging was done at night by a gang of low men surrounded by lewd women, who loafed in the daytime and prowled around at night, and that the Smiths were the worst of the gang. (19)

In addition, Joseph, Jr. and Emma had left Harmony, Pennsylvania, on short notice in 1830, perhaps because, as has been speculated, Emma's cousin Hiel Lewis had accused Joseph of unsavory conduct with women, including an attempt to seduce one Eliza Winters (20). In response to criticism of his moral character, Joseph once even admitted to being "subject to passion" (21).

Aside from such vague and ill-documented references, however, no specific sexual conduct is recorded until Joseph's midtwenties, when a serial pattern of sexual relationships with women other than his wife Emma begins to be documented. Ironically, most of this documentation derives from efforts of the main body of Mormonism itself to discredit the claim of the Reorganized faction that Joseph had been monogamous. However, that motive, in turn, has tended to favor a historical record highlighting only those relationships falling into a specifically sanctioned framework.

---

[1] A sizable number of sworn affidavits was collected in 1833 from more than 100 individuals who had known the Joseph Smith family in upstate New York. Compiled originally by Philastus Hurlbut, an excommunicated Mormon and enemy of the Prophet, they were published by Eber D. Howe in 1834. The affidavits generally supported the materials contained in the court record and the contemporary editorials of the *Palmyra Register*.

The second fully documented extramarital liaison of Joseph was with a teenager who, like Nancy Marinda Johnson three years previously, was living for a time under the same roof in the Kirtland, Ohio, area. Fannie Alger was a charming 17-year-old orphan girl whom Emma had taken into the family home in 1835. Rumors of Joseph's affair with Fannie were most painful to Emma, who was understandably possessive of her dashing husband and wished to protect his dignified position within his church. Confirmation of those rumors was provided when a suspicious friend (and likely Emma herself) spied on the two in the hay loft of the barn and witnessed their lovemaking. *The Book of Mormon* transcriptionist Oliver Cowdery, bitterly offended by Joseph's "dirty, nasty, filthy affair" (22), angrily confronted the prophet, beginning a schism between the two that would lead to Cowdery's excommunication from the church three years later. After several months of the affair, Fannie was "unable to conceal the consequences of her celestial relation with the prophet" (23), and Emma drove the gravid orphan out of the house and out of town (24).

Joseph's third known extramarital relationship began three years later in 1838, again with a woman living in the same household. Lucinda Pendleton Morgan Harris had been married to William Morgan, the famous anti-Masonic crusader who had been murdered in upstate New York just before the writing of *The Book of Mormon*. Lucinda had then married George Harris, and the couple had become involved in the growing church. Joseph's relationship with her in the Mormon community of Far West, Missouri, occurred while Joseph was boarding with the couple. Lucinda Harris later corroborated the nature of the relationship herself in an 1842 conversation with an indignant married woman whom Joseph had just unsuccessfully propositioned. The latter woman, Mrs. Sarah Pratt, related, "When Joseph had made his dastardly attempt on me, I went to Mrs. Harris to unbosom my grief to her. To my utter astonishment, she said, laughing heartily: 'How foolish you are! I don't see anything so horrible in it. Why, I am his mistress since four years'" (25).

Interestingly, the married status of Lucinda Harris was to become the rule rather than the exception in what is known of the

early portion of the succeeding series of Joseph's sexual conquests. Although no one knows for certain how many such affairs
Joseph had during his short adult life, Brodie was able to document forty-eight from various records (26), and Stanley Ivins esti-
mated the number to be possibly as many as eighty-four (27).
Except for the young women boarding in his home, Joseph provided none of them with any of the traditional spousal support of
food, clothing, or shelter. In Brodie's list, ten of the first thirteen
were already married to someone else at the time of Joseph's liaisons with them. Nevertheless, Joseph was not always so discrimi-
nating. As Mrs. Sarah Pratt, in her sworn affidavit, relates,

> I have told you that the prophet Joseph used to frequent
> houses of ill-fame. Mrs. White, a very pretty and attractive
> woman, once confessed to me that she made a business of it
> to be hospitable to the captains of the Mississippi steam-
> boats. She told me that Joseph had made her acquaintance
> very soon after his arrival in Nauvoo, and that he had visited
> her dozens of times . . .
>
> Next door to my house was a house of bad reputation.
> One single woman lived there, not very attractive. She used
> to be visited by people from Carthage whenever they came
> to Nauvoo. Joseph used to come on horseback, ride up to
> the house and tie his horse to a tree, many of which stood
> before the house. Then he would enter the house of the
> woman from the back. I have seen him do this repeatedly.
> (28)

That Joseph Smith, Jr. had a voracious sexual appetite that
seemed to demand multiple conquests is in itself not unprece-
dented for a charismatic leader. What *is* unique is the superstructure of rationalization that he devised to justify his conduct to
society and to himself. Joseph proclaimed a sea-change in the very
institution of marriage itself. His identification with the Old Testament character Jacob has already been noted in Joseph's selection
of the name "Laban" (Jacob's deceitful father-in-law in the Old
Testament) for the repugnant evil-father representation of *The
Book of Mormon*'s opening pages. The fact that Jacob did not
need to content himself with the homely Leah as his sole wife

seemed to confirm to Joseph that he, too, had no need to chafe under the restriction of monogamy when there were so many Rachels around whom he could also take to the marital bed. Joseph frequently referred to his new system of multiple wives as "the blessing of Jacob," though he occasionally dropped the names of Abraham, Moses, Isaac, David, and Solomon as well.

Rationalizing his promiscuous sexual conduct in a convincing way would be vitally important for Joseph if he wished to succeed as a saintly leader over a flock drawn from humble folk with traditionalist mores. As he was seemingly driven by his pattern of sexual behavior, this conduct somehow had to be reconciled within the framework of his religious status as prophet of God—no mean feat. Joseph appears to have recognized this incongruity very early when his ambitions about a church were only in his imagination. In *The Book of Mormon* he pointedly defines plural marriage as a legitimate Old Testament sacrament and then proceeds to forbid it to the Nephites:

> Behold, David and Solomon truly had many wives and concubines, which thing was abominable before me, saith the Lord. . . . Wherefore, I, the Lord God, will not suffer that this people shall do like unto them of old . . . for there shall not any man among you have save it be one wife; and concubines he shall have none. (Jacob 2, p. 127)

But in the very next verse, Joseph makes it clear that things may become quite different in the latter days: "For if I will, saith the Lord of Hosts, raise up seed unto me, I will command my people: otherwise, they shall hearken unto these things" (Jacob 2, p. 127).

The implication that God might override at any time his restrictive rules for the Nephites is unmistakable. Thus was the issue opened from the moment of the birth of Mormonism, and thus had it undoubtedly been incubating in some form well before the formal religious conception. Although the new marital order would not be given the ultimate imprimatur of a written revelation through Joseph Smith, Jr. until July 12, 1843, the prophet had by that time practiced its tenets for many years and had selectively shared them with chosen members of his priesthood.

Several pieces of reliable evidence date Joseph's embrace of the formal principle of polygamy as early as 1831, in the very earliest days of his church. On July 17, 1831, Joseph proclaimed a revelation to seven elders in western Missouri:

> For it is my will, that in time, ye should take unto you wives of the Lamanites and Nephites that their posterity may become white, delightsome and just, for even now their females are more virtuous than the gentiles. (29)

A note appended to W. W. Phelps's handwritten copy of the revelation adds the following:

> About three years after this was given, I asked brother Joseph, privately, how "we," that were mentioned in the revelation could take wives of the "natives" as we were all married men? He replied instantly, "In the same manner that Abraham took Hagar and Keturah; that Jacob took Rachel, Bilhah and Zilpah; by revelation—the saints of the Lord are always directed by revelation." (30)

It is likely that some reference to divine sanction accompanied each of Joseph's sexual relationships from the time of the founding of the church, although Mrs. Sarah Pratt thought otherwise:

> You should bear in mind that Joseph did not think of a marriage or sealing ceremony for many years. He used to state to his intended victims, as he did to me: "God does not care if we have a good time, if only other people do not know it." He only introduced a marriage ceremony when he had found out that he could not get certain women without it. I think Louisa Beaman was the first of this kind. If any woman, like me, opposed his wishes, he used to say: "Be silent, or I shall ruin your character. My character must be sustained in the interest of the church." (31)

Divine sanction or no, rumors of secret polygamous relationships were attributed to Mormon enclaves from the earliest days of the church and dogged the movement wherever it went. Because this sort of accusation is an unusual one per se, even among the frontier's several revolutionary social movements of which Joseph's church was but one, these persistent, sequential claims by Mormonism's detractors of plural wives in several widely separated locations give tacit validity to the allegations and focus the responsibility for the practice on one man.

The practice of plural marriage under Joseph Smith's leadership reached its dangerous apogee in the Mormon community of Nauvoo, Illinois, in the early 1840s—dangerous because the vast majority of the more than ten thousand faithful and devout Latter-day Saints living in what was at the time the largest city in Illinois incredibly knew virtually nothing of the existence of such a practice. Joseph had correctly predetermined that he would not be able to hold the loyalty of his rank and file if knowledge of his own habitual sexual practices became widespread. Yet, seemingly unable to abandon his promiscuous conduct, he must somehow justify it to the loyal and faithful Mormon women whom he approached, and often to their husbands, from whom he diverted the women's fealties. A prophet could not long remain a prophet if tagged as a libertine.

It was a measure of Joseph's grandiosity that he felt fully justified as the Lord's mouthpiece to override the fundamental societal convention of monogamous marriage rather than to alter his own habits. His very boldness in pursuing his course and the carefully measured pace with which he shared the blessing of Jacob with his confidants bought time for his sexual conduct to continue and for him to gain the tolerance of most of his immediate circle of associates.

Unlike Mrs. Sarah Pratt, most of the women Joseph approached seemed receptive to his entreaties. He was, after all, the prophet—the infallible voice of God on earth, the reason for their sharing this enchanted island in society, the brilliant translator of ancient languages, the founder of the restored church, the fiery inspirator at the pulpit, and the healer of the sick. He was, in addition, a sexy man. He stood six feet tall and had a robust build, youthful appearance, and handsome, deep-set blue eyes. A strikingly pale countenance and light brown hair framed his contagious smile, and his affable charm and lively wit were said to dominate every gathering. In the ever-increasing isolation of the Mormon community, made all the more stark by the growing hostility roundabout, the need to rely on the prophet's personal guidance grew daily as contact with mainstream America dwindled.

In this context an enthralling divine revelation described in confidence to a flattered and worshipful admirer during a quiet walk might well have evoked a breath-stopping effect, especially if delivered in utmost secrecy. For a woman to hesitate—to deflect the invitation—would have been to deny the divine infallibility of the prophet. To accept would have meant violation of a basic taboo, and there were no disinterested third parties to consult for guidance in this shocking matter. Joseph frequently asked his startled companions to pray for guidance or a sign, excusing himself tenderly. The troubled nights that would follow for his prospective mates would more often than not work to his advantage. The target of his affections was often a "church widow," enduring loneliness after Joseph had sent her husband to Canada or England in pursuit of converts. Or her search for a more meaningful life might have drawn her toward the enchanting promise of the Mormon kingdom, leaving her less mystical husband in the reality of the farm and its debts. Whatever the reason, the answer to Joseph's tender entreaties was in the affirmative with sufficient frequency that the prophet's celestial family grew apace.

A clear example of Joseph's skill in applying such pressure is demonstrated in the description of his proposition to naive 17-year-old Lucy Walker, who was living in the prophet's house. Joseph, then 37, approached her during Emma's absence with a brief description of "celestial marriage" and then, by her account, stated, "I have no flattering words to offer. It is a command of God to you. I will give you until tomorrow to decide this matter. If you reject this message the gate will be closed forever against you." When she hesitated, Joseph approached and pronounced, "God Almighty bless you. You shall have testimony that you can never deny. I will tell you what it shall be. It shall be that joy and peace that you never knew." The aftermath of shock and insomnia were soon overpowering to the young girl, and none too soon. Emma returned the day after the childlike Lucy had experienced in the wee hours her "irresistible testimony of the truth of plural marriage" (32) and relinquished her virginity.

The general reaction of the men with whom Joseph confided his revelation on celestial marriage was similarly troubled, but the outcome—that of agonizing approval—was similar. Joseph's lips would breathe not a word of it, of course, to any who were not among his most trusted and loyal priesthood.

These men of God were usually introduced to the principle with a more convoluted theological schema than were the women. The entire community of men and gods (yes, gods) was one of progression, Joseph taught. As men are now, the Father once was; and as the Father is, man may become. Thus, a kind of literal pursuit of "father's" status seems to have found its way into Joseph's eschatology. If one was blessed by the sacraments (as administered through God's prophet), celestial glory could be obtained. One could expand one's glory and one's personal kingdom with an ever-greater increase in offspring until they were as numberless as the stars in the sky. This would be made possible through the taking of more and more wives, all of whom would remain ever faithful and continue after death to give spiritual and sexual pleasure and to bear children (if they had been properly sealed to the man on earth through the prophet). Thus a man might "seal" himself to two or more living wives in the same manner that he would marry them sequentially if one were to die and leave him a widower. Furthermore, Joseph explained, although a woman might already be married to one man "for time" on earth, she might legitimately choose to be sealed to another "for eternity" to become a part of the latter's celestial kingdom, all the while not violating the marriage code or committing adultery.

And, of course, if the eternal husband were to be permitted to enjoy his celestial wife's sexual favors in the hereafter, there was no legitimate reason to deny them in this short temporal existence either. Strict adherence to the prophet's revealed requirements would mean great eschatological glories to be won, greater and more exotic than had ever been dreamed in any traditional Western religion. (And again, achieving that status that "father" possessed would be done through sexual means, a universal wish of the male child.) Any awkwardness experienced by a devout

Mormon husband when explaining this new order to his traditional wife, Joseph clarified, merely reflected the need for some
resolve and readjustment in order to restore these Old Testament
sacraments. Indeed, the very difficulty in accepting the new practice, Joseph went on, was proof of its divine origin as a test of faith.
Only those who could accept the difficult challenge could enjoy
its fruits. To his most loyal priesthood, Joseph offered forbidden
pleasures and incomparable dreams.

Initially, as with the women, Joseph carefully selected his male
confidants one by one. He knew with whom he dared share his
new order and with whom he dared not. But because every disclosure carried the substantial risk of public dissemination, there
had to be sufficient reason to expand the tiny circle of cognoscenti in the secret order. A bold step was taken by Joseph on
April 5, 1841, when the first written recording of a sealing ceremony took place with the prophet's marriage to the lovely
26-year-old Louisa Beaman (who was mentioned in Sarah Pratt's
affidavit, as noted earlier on p. 176). As Louisa had been boarding
with her married older sister at the time, Joseph had evidently felt
it prudent first to instruct Louisa's brother-in-law, Elder Joseph
Bates Noble, in the secret mysteries of the newly restored kingdom. After several sleepless nights and fasting, Noble had accepted the new order with some enthusiasm. With this source of
the maiden's potential protection neutralized, Joseph then spoke
with Mrs. Noble, who agonized and finally also granted a troubled
assent to her sister's hand. Only then did Joseph gently approach
Louisa—with success. A swift promotion to bishop followed for
Noble, along with an invitation to move from an outlying village
into Nauvoo. Noble was then granted the ultimate honor: he was
personally chosen to officiate at the first-ever recorded sealing
ceremony—that for his sister-in-law and the prophet. The risks
had paid off as Joseph was growing ever bolder in his selection of
sexual partners.

But the reticence experienced by Joseph's intended sexual
partners and by his priesthood confidants was nothing compared
with the intransigent resistance to the new order posed by his
wife Emma. She was intensely jealous of his affections and sensed
the need to preserve the dignity and respectability of his office in

the church. She furthermore felt a duty to her sons not to subject them to the sort of disgrace to which she knew their father's conduct would inevitably condemn them during their adult lives. Joseph had, in addition, maintained his dashing youthful countenance while she, older than he at the outset, was showing the physical ravages of multiparity and the uncommon emotional stresses and dangers of her eventful existence.

What is known of the private interactions and conversations of the couple concerning the issue suggests a kind of seething standoff. She bitterly resented the rumors of her husband's dalliances and apparently badgered him endlessly about the hushed stories. He evidently responded with denials, which she, in turn, publicly proclaimed in order to reinforce the standard against which she and the vast majority of the church would measure him. She presided over the Nauvoo Female Relief Society, speaking out strongly against plural marriage and attempting to establish a network of informants against her husband and his associates over the practice.

Needless to say, Joseph took elaborate precautions to avoid any possibility of discovery by Emma during his liaisons. An example of his stealth is seen in his August 1842 letter to his recently sealed 17-year-old plural wife Sarah Ann Whitney and her approving parents:

> The nights are very pleasant, indeed, all three of you can come and See me in the fore part of the night, let Brother Whitney come a little a head and nock at the south East corner of the house, at the window; it is next to the cornfield; I have a room entirely by myself, the whole matter can be attended to with the most perfect safty. The only thing to be careful of, is to find out when Emma comes, then you can not be Safe, but when she is not here, there is the most perfect safty. . . . Burn this letter as soon as you read it. keep all locked up in your breasts, my life depends upon it one thing I want to see you for, is to git the fulness of my blessing Sealed upon our heads. . . . I think Emma wont come to-night if she dont, dont fail to come to night. (33)

By the spring of 1843, Joseph had tipped the balance in the stalemate slightly in his favor. Emma had finally capitulated by

agreeing to accommodate more "wives," but only if she could select them. The nod went grudgingly to Emily and Eliza Partridge,
19- and 23-year-old sisters living with the Smith family under Joseph's
guardianship after the death of their bishop father (whose estate
was much diminished after Joseph had borrowed $10,000 from
it). Both sisters were formally sealed to the prophet on May 11,
1843, with Emma's half-hearted assent. (What Emma did not
know was that her eager husband had already married both
young women two months before without her imprimatur.) In addition, Emma agreed to Joseph's marriage to the 17- and 19-year-
old Lawrence sisters, also orphaned and living with the Smith
family under Joseph's guardianship. The four marriages, however, did not settle the argument, but merely shifted its focus to
ceasing the practice. Emma had, in the meantime, shortly driven
the Partridge sisters from her home with her bitter jealousy.

The assent to her husband's polygamy had been wrested from
Emma by a form of spiritual extortion. Joseph had preached in
early 1843 that women would soon be permitted to participate in
the "endowment ceremonies" (to be described in Chapter 8). He
had taught Emma that the endowment was necessary for "exalta-
tion" in the next world. Yet he refused to permit her participation
in the endowment ceremonies until she was obedient and
granted him plural wives. Five days after Emma witnessed Joseph's
sealing ceremony to the Partridge sisters, she was sealed to Joseph for "time and all eternity" and was initiated into the endowment three months later (34).

The talented young poet Eliza Snow also lived under Joseph's
roof for a time, serving Emma in her duties and tutoring the Smith
children as "Aunt Eliza." Joseph was patient in his courtship of her
and sealed her to himself only after a flowery prelude, made necessary by her strong early resistance to the new marriage order.
Since Emma trusted Eliza deeply, she had tried to enlist the poet's
assistance in spying on Joseph in his relations with other women.
Soon the prophet had impregnated both women, and concealment became impossible. When Joseph momentarily embraced
Eliza one morning in the hall, Emma unexpectedly emerged from
her bedroom and guessed at once the nature of the deception.
She attacked Eliza with a broomstick in sudden ferocious anger.

The defenseless Eliza tripped and tumbled down the flight of stairs behind her, still under vicious attack from the enraged Emma. Though Joseph came to Eliza's aid, it was too late. She lost her baby and was never to conceive again.

It was Joseph's brother Hyrum, by now with several wives of his own, who conceived the logical solution to Joseph's troubles with Emma. If Joseph would only have the revelation on celestial marriage written down, Hyrum offered, "I will take it and read it to Emma, and I believe I can convince her of its truth, and you will hereafter have peace." Joseph smiled and responded, "You do not know Emma as well as I do" (35). After a short exchange, Joseph dubiously agreed and dictated the final revelation of his life to Elder William Clayton, his personal clerk, on July 12, 1843. Rich in Joseph's familiar imagery, the lengthy document read, in part, as follows:

> Verily, thus saith the Lord unto you, my servant Joseph, that inasmuch as you have enquired of my hand, to know and understand wherein I, the Lord, justified my servants Abraham, Isaac and Jacob; as also Moses, David and Solomon, my servants, as touching the principle and doctrine of their having many wives and concubines:
>
> Behold . . . I reveal unto you a new and an everlasting covenant.
>
> And again, verily I say unto you, if a man marry a wife by my word . . . and it is sealed unto them by . . . [Joseph Smith] . . . [they] shall inherit thrones, kingdoms, principalities, and powers, dominions, all heights and depths . . .
>
> Then shall they be gods, because they have no end.
>
> Abraham received promises concerning his seed, and of the fruit of his loins—from whose loins ye are, namely, my servant Joseph . . .
>
> Go ye, therefore, and do the works of Abraham; enter ye into my law, and ye shall be saved . . .
>
> God commanded Abraham, and Sarah gave Hagar to Abraham to wife. . . .
>
> Was Abraham, therefore, under condemnation? . . . Nay; for I, the Lord, commanded it. . . .
>
> Abraham received concubines, and they bare him children . . . as Isaac also, and Jacob . . .

David also received many wives and concubines, as also Solomon and Moses my servants.

If a man receive a wife in the new and everlasting covenant, and if she be with another man, and I have not appointed unto her by the holy anointing, she hath committed adultery, and shall be destroyed . . .

. . . if she hath not committed adultery, but is innocent . . . then shall you have power, by the power of my Holy Priesthood, to take her, and give her unto him that hath not committed adultery . . .

And again, verily I say unto you my servant Joseph, that whatsoever you give on earth, and to whomsoever you give any one on earth, by my word, and according to my law, it shall be visited with blessings . . .

And let mine handmaid, Emma Smith, receive all those that have been given unto my servant, Joseph . . .

. . . and I command my handmaid, Emma Smith, to abide and cleave unto my servant Joseph, and to none else . . . for I am the Lord thy God, and will destroy her, if she abide not in my law . . .

. . . and I will bless [Joseph] and multiply him, and give unto him an hundred fold in this world, of fathers and mothers, brothers and sisters, houses and lands, wives and children, and crowns of eternal lives in the eternal worlds.

If any man espouse a virgin, and desire to espouse another, and the first give her consent; and if he espouse the second, and they are virgins, and have vowed to no other man, then is he justified . . .

. . . and if he have ten virgins given unto him by this law, he cannot commit adultery, for they belong to him. . . .

But if one or either of the ten virgins after she is espoused shall be with another man she has committed adultery. (36)

Hyrum returned from his presentation of the revelation to Emma much chastised, admitting, "that he had never received a more severe talking to in his life, that Emma was very bitter and full of resentment and anger," to which Joseph quietly replied, "I told you you did not know Emma as well as I did" (37).

Initially frightened by the written revelation, Emma confided to Apostle William Law, "The revelation says I must submit or be destroyed. Well, I guess I'll have to submit" (38). However, soon regaining her courage, she again went on the offensive, with tears and threats to leave her husband. Finally he relinquished the hated document to her, whereupon she triumphantly burned it in the fireplace. But as if to mock the paragraphs of the revelation relating directly to her, God did not destroy Emma Smith.

In the future and in her own way, Emma would have her revenge. She may or may not have known that she had assisted as midwife at the birth of at least one child Joseph had fathered (39). She later would bitterly denounce polygamy, proclaiming to her son Joseph III, "He had no other wife but me" (40), thus branding as immoral those other women who had shared their beds with her husband. She would teach her sons that their deceased father had been faithful and monogamous, surrounded by iniquitous men performing evil and licentious acts in his name. She would refuse to recognize the church's chosen leadership after her husband's death and would refuse to join the migration westward. And she would remarry, but to a non-Mormon.

Joseph's careful nurturing of his plural marriage doctrine was bent into convoluted turns by his relationship with a new arrival in Nauvoo in mid-1840, a man with whom he shared not only the same age but an equivalent narcissism and sexual appetite as well. Dr. John C. Bennett was quartermaster general of the Illinois militia, secretary of the Illinois Medical Society, a Methodist lay minister, and an authority on obstetrical matters. His skill in oratory and writing, his political acumen, his knowledge of civil engineering, and his military experience permitted Joseph to obtain a charter for his city, build and train a large personal militia, curry favor with both political parties, and plot out the physical blueprint of Nauvoo. Having originally flattered Joseph with a series of introductory letters, Bennett had risen within a few months of his arrival to become the first mayor of Nauvoo, chancellor of the new Nauvoo University, major general of the Nauvoo Legion (Joseph was lieutenant general), and "assistant president" of the church.

It was in the sexual arena, however, that the most critical feature of their relationship existed, for better and for worse. Bennett had perhaps been drawn to Nauvoo by the rumors concerning polygamy. He had previously deserted his wife and family in Morgan County, Ohio, and was said to be dashing with women. He was a frequenter of the not-so-clandestine brothels in town and had soon charmed numerous prominent women of Nauvoo society by his dark features and loquacious manner. As one of Joseph's intimates, he learned and practiced the blessing of Jacob along with apostles Heber Kimball and Brigham Young, the latter having become over several years Joseph's most powerful religious ally. But Bennett was not particularly religious and seems to have paid little homage to the eternal aspects of the sealing or to his personal progression toward building a celestial kingdom. Many seductions evidently took place without any pretense of a sealing ceremony.

Bennett was evidently of inestimable value to Joseph, however, for his gynecologic skills. As the ultimate consequences of the blessing of Jacob were blessed events, the doctor's talents were periodically solicited. Bennett had even promised to each of his own consorts that he could abort any pregnancy resulting from their union. Sarah Pratt stated of Bennett concerning an occasion when he had ridden to her house to retrieve a borrowed book:

> While giving Bennett his book, I observed that he held something in the left sleeve of his coat. Bennett smiled and said: "Oh, a little job for Joseph: one of his women is in trouble." Saying this, he took the thing out of his left sleeve. It was a pretty long instrument of a kind I had never seen before. It seemed to be of steel and was crooked at one end. I heard afterward that the operation had been performed; that the woman was very sick, and that Joseph was very much afraid that she might die, but she recovered. (41)

But Nauvoo was soon to prove too small to harbor both Joseph Smith, Jr. and John C. Bennett. Not surprisingly, they broke over the affections of a woman. Nancy Rigdon was the beautiful 19-year-old daughter of Sidney Rigdon, one of Joseph's earliest stalwarts in the faith and now his First Counselor. Both prophet and doctor were unusually solicitous of the young woman, with her dignified and refined manner. As Joseph had watched her grow to maturity over the past eleven years, he was not amused by her new admiration for the dapper Bennett. Wishing in turn to

thwart Joseph's designs, Bennett forewarned Nancy of the prophet's notions of celestial marriage and suggested she be on her
guard. Knowing that he had little to no chance of persuading Nancy's devout, Puritanical father of the new marriage order, Joseph
arranged a private liaison with the girl through the aid of an older
woman of the church, a member of the "Mothers in Israel," whose
complicity in the new order often took such a catalytic role. Nancy
responded to his entreaties with affronted anger and threatened
to expose his actions to the entire city unless he released her.
Joseph dictated the following letter to her a day later:

> Happiness is the object and design of our existence, and
> will be the end thereof, if we pursue the path that leads to it
> . . . but we cannot keep all the commandments without first
> knowing them. . . . That which is wrong under one circum-
> stance, may be, and often is, right under another. . . . What-
> ever god requires is right, no matter what it is, although we
> may not see the reason thereof till long after the events tran-
> spire. . . . So with Solomon; first he asked wisdom, and god
> gave it him, and with it every desire of his heart; even things
> which might be considered abominable to all who under-
> stand the order of Heaven only in part. . . . Blessings of-
> fered, but rejected, are no longer blessings.
>   . . . for all things shall be made known unto them in mine
> own due time, and in the end they shall have joy. (42)

Indignantly, Nancy told her father about Joseph's proposition
and his views on celestial wifery, and she showed him the letter.
Sidney Rigdon angrily confronted Joseph with Nancy's story of attempted seduction. The prophet denied the allegations until confronted with the letter. He then broke down and confessed but
stated that he had done it all merely as a test of Nancy's purity and
virtue.

Joseph had no choice; Bennett had to go. Nevertheless, the
prophet knew the doctor had the knowledge and the rhetorical
skill to do him great harm. After a couple of halting attempts to
silence Bennett with threats, Joseph excommunicated him. Immediately Bennett turned on Joseph from outside Nauvoo, publishing lurid, exaggerated accounts of the political and military

goals of Mormonism, of the treachery and fanaticism of the leadership, and of the moral and sexual depravity of Joseph and the priesthood. Names were named and affidavits were quoted. Joseph's
letter to Nancy Rigdon was published.

The counterattack had to be fierce and frantic, as the devout
members of the Mormon community suddenly were confronted
with news that shook the very roots of their faith. Joseph fought
back by blaming all of the moral decay on Bennett himself, and all
the illegitimate infants of Nauvoo suddenly adopted the same pa-
ternity. Joseph angrily denied all of the stories of celestial wives,
and all of the cadre, both men and women, who knew and participated fell in behind him with sworn affidavits and bitter denuncia-
tions of any such practices. Joseph did not break, and neither did
his disciples—this time.

But as Joseph evidently had no capacity to abandon his driven
sexual behavior, he crafted the ultimate trial balloon to test public
acceptance of the clandestine sacrament. Joseph appointed Ud-
ney Jacob to select Old Testament passages pertaining to polygamy and to assemble them into a persuasive pamphlet on the
subject. Jacob complied and added a lengthy defense of polygamy
as an alternative to an unhappy marriage. How much the statement is a reflection of Joseph's own personal situation is conjec-
tural. The pamphlet, "The Peace Maker," set forth, in part, the
following:

> Adam was enslaved by the woman, and SO ARE WE. . . .
> What, although a woman is not known to be an adulteress,
> yet she may be a PERFECT DEVIL to her husband, train him
> in the most imperious manner, despise him in her heart,
> abuse him before his children, drive him like a menial slave
> where she pleases; and he must tamely submit to the un-
> godly law of his wife, must hug the serpent to his bosom,
> and love her as he does his own body! Impossible, and de-
> grading to the nature of man . . .
>
> But suppose a man (that has already a wife) entice a
> maid; how then could he marry her? If a man entice a maid
> that is not betrothed, and lie with her, he shall surely endow
> her to be his wife. There is no condition that can justify him
> in refusing to marry her . . .

> There is no positive law of God against a man's marrying
> Leah and Rachel both. . . . To God only are men account-
> able in this matter, and not to their wives . . . by depriving
> him of the RIGHT OF MARRYING MORE THAN ONE WIFE,
> you totally annihilate his power of peaceable government
> over a woman, and deprive the family of its lawful and nec-
> essary head . . .
> POLYGAMY regulated by the law of God as illustrated in this
> book could not possibly produce one crime; neither could it
> injure any human being. The stupidity of modern Christian
> nations upon this subject is horribly astonishing. (43)

Although "J. Smith" was listed as the printer of the tract, the
public outrage against the pamphlet was so shrill, coming on the
heels of the Bennett mess, that the prophet had to scapegoat Ud-
ney Jacob and brand the publication as an outrage in a carefully
worded newspaper notice:

> There was a book printed at my office a short time since,
> written by Udney H[.] Jacob, on marriage, without my
> knowledge; and had I been apprised of it, I should not have
> printed it; not that I am opposed to any man enjoying his
> privileges, but I do not wish to have my name associated
> with the authors, in such an unmeaning rigmarole of non-
> sense, folly and trash.
>
> Joseph Smith (44)

In his disavowal Joseph restricted his condemnation to the pamphlet itself, wishing not to have his name associated with such
a publication that had aroused such scandal. The trial balloon had
crashed.

Brodie has divided her own count of Joseph's forty-eight plural wives into three general groups (45). The first group comprised more than a dozen women, most of whom were married,
who were "sealed" to Joseph prior to Bennett's departure. The
second group was largely composed of women of the principal
leadership of the Nauvoo Female Relief Society, a charitable organization that, as noted above, was beginning to snoop, under
Emma's inquisitive leadership, after the rumors of iniquity in the
city following Bennett's expulsion. The prophet, to state the mat-

ter indelicately, seemed to be buying protection against his wife. The third, and final, group comprised mostly young, single women, some no more than 15 years of age. Evidently, some of these women in the final year were sealed to Joseph at the rate of three or more per month.

Joseph was not entirely unselfish in his acquisition of spiritual wives. With thousands of women living in and around Nauvoo, even one as prodigious as he could not share the blessing of Jacob with even a creditable fraction. He would have known implicitly that no contingent of his priesthood, much less his rank and file, would accept through faith and loyalty any sanctioning of his new sexual order so long as it applied only to Joseph himself. But, on the other hand, by the necessity of gradually sharing the benefits of the sacrament with his associates, he knew that certain kinds of complexities must inevitably arise. The episode with Nancy Rigdon demonstrated how the danger of rivalry for feminine affections could cause friction, or worse, between two ardent suitors. There was obviously the potential for the appearance of competition that would inevitably take root as more men entered the fraternity of celestial kingdoms, or what Joseph called the "Everlasting Covenant." And the wider was the participation, the less would be the security and the confidentiality of the sacrament from the main body of parishioners (and from the unquenchable curiosity of Emma), to say nothing of the increasingly hostile non-Mormon community around Nauvoo. Explosive instability would be the inevitable consequence of these necessary compromises the prophet chose in his decision to rationalize his sexual conduct rather than to change it.

But was this indeed a conscious decision? What were the forces at play in Joseph's mind that would tilt Mormon history itself in this socially repugnant direction? Why didn't he simply choose to behave within the accepted limits of society's sexual norms? With the well-earned and steadfast loyalty of thousands of followers, why did he find it so hard to grow into the role model he knew his flock expected? The theology, the organization, and the body of socioreligious experience he had created were easily sufficient in and of themselves to ensure the continued mushrooming of a vast religious empire. Why would he insist on adding this unnecessary, treacherous, and suicidal appendage?

The answers to these questions must lie, as is always the case with perverse behavior, in the mist of Joseph's childhood, for they can have no basis in the rational and logical sectors of his mind. Whether the number of sexual conquests was forty-eight, eighty-four, or two hundred, something was at work in Joseph's mind that compelled him to degrade women into sexual objects and that prevented him from enjoying the true intimacy of a one-on-one relationship that most adults ultimately achieve. Joseph's unusual sexual behavior appears to have been highly repetitive in its pattern and compulsive in its execution. He likely could not have altered it in a lasting way any more than his father could have stopped dreaming of finding treasures in the earth. Joseph Smith, Jr. was indeed following orders, but were they from above or from within?

What were those orders and what was the nature of the command? Joseph Smith, Jr. provides the answer himself. Lorenzo Snow, one of Joseph's successors as president of the Latter-day Saint Church in Utah, swore of polygamy's origin:

> President Joseph Smith said he wished to have some private talk with me, and requested me to walk out with him. . . . He there and then explained to me the doctrine of plurality of wives; he said that the Lord had revealed it unto him, and commanded him to have women sealed to him as wives; that he foresaw the trouble that would follow, and sought to turn away from the commandment; *that an angel from heaven then appeared before him with a drawn sword, threatening him with destruction unless he went forward and obeyed the commandment.* (46) (emphasis added)

Snow's sister Eliza, the poet and plural wife of Joseph, describes her brother's recollections of Joseph's apparition with more threatening imagery. Joseph had

> hesitated and deferred from time to time, until an angel of God stood by him with a drawn sword and told him that, unless he moved forward and established plural marriage, his

Priesthood would be taken from him and he should be destroyed! . . . (47)

Benjamin F. Johnson, later the Patriarch of the Church in Utah, swore of Joseph's conversation with him in 1843:

[Joseph] also visited my mother at her residence in Macedonio and taught her in my hearing the doctrine of celestial marriage, declaring that an angel appeared unto him with a drawn sword, threatening to slay him if he did not proceed to fulfill the law that had been given to him. (48)

Johnson related a second 1843 incident in which Joseph's brother Hyrum told him,

Now Benjamin, you must not be afraid of this new doctrine, for it is all right. You know Brother Hyrum don't get carried away by worldly things, and he fought this principle until the Lord showed him it was true. I know that Joseph was commanded to take more wives, and he waited until an angel with drawn sword stood before him and declared that if he longer delayed fulfilling that command that he would slay him. (49)

Joseph gave an even more detailed description of the irresistible force to one of his more reluctant sexual conquests, thereby suggesting in the process that the powerful visage was more than an occasional visitor in his thoughts concerning the subject of plural marriage. Mary Elizabeth Rollins Lightner, married to a non-Mormon, had been an object of Joseph's desires in 1831 and again in 1834. In 1842, as he pressed toward the ultimate consummation of his longings, he described to her the same uninvited apparition that drove his actions. She later swore that

[i]n 1834 [Joseph] was commanded to take me for a wife. I was a thousand miles from him. He got afraid. The angel came to him three times, the last time with a drawn sword and threatened his life. (50)

Unlike ordinary dreams, those that are repetitive are unique in psychic life, for they are nearly always playbacks of frightening experiences that have actually happened (51). It should come as no surprise that Joseph should have experienced frequent nightmares about his childhood operations, for the imagery described in these passages can hardly relate to anything else. But why should these frightening images of Dr. Nathan Smith in any way be linked in Joseph's thought processes to the subject of plural marriage? Could this be a rare instance in which a recurring dream might be of value for the study of history?

Before attempting to sort out the reason for this linkage, it must be shown that the content of the sworn statements themselves are indeed images related to Joseph's surgical procedures. It will be recalled that in dreams—and daydreams, for that matter—kings, presidents, angels, judges, policemen, and the like are usually representations of the father. The fused angel image of his father and Dr. Nathan Smith should have been a powerful and threatening dream apparition for Joseph for all the reasons previously presented. The fact that this father-image carried a drawn sword makes any alternative explanation for this personage unlikely. Mrs. Lightner further related that the angel "came to him three times." (How many operations?)

Finally, there is Joseph's affect, his emotion toward the angel: that of extreme terror. The angel is a powerfully punitive, male creature in the dream. He is there not to love, not to assist, but to command and threaten. And if the angel's will should not be done, what would be the consequence? Lorenzo Snow remembered "destruction"; Mrs. Lightner remembered that the angel "threatened his life," and Benjamin Johnson remembered that the angel threatened to "slay him." But the poet Eliza Snow recalled the full sanction against the man she called husband: "his Priesthood would be taken from him and he should be destroyed." In the symbols of his dream Joseph would lose his priesthood—his potency.

And why was this to happen? For what terrible guilty act was this awful punishment to be meted out? In the dissociated memory of his childhood it had been linked to his age-appropriate fantasy of forbidden sexuality. But why now was it all reversed? Why was the angel there to emasculate Joseph if he did *not* establish plural marriage? If he did *not* rescue Elizabeth Lightner from Adam Lightner?

The work of psychoanalyst Otto Fenichel offers one plausible explanation. Fenichel points out that the *fears* a child feels when experiencing erotic sensations may become a lasting part of his world of sexuality (52). Usually these defenses against fear, called phobias, produce behavior that *avoids* what is feared when some *punishment* may threaten.[2]

However, some individuals react paradoxically by actually *seeking out* those situations that they fear, or even developing a *preference* for them. When individuals thus compulsively seek out a formerly feared situation again and again, it is called a *counter-phobia*. But because powerful emotions continue in counter-phobic behavior, people with counter-phobias are as anxiety-ridden over their *search* for something as phobic individuals are over their avoidance. Thus, says Fenichel,

> The "counter-phobic attitude" . . . cannot . . . be overcome if the activity against which it is directed has a hidden sexual significance. . . . He seeks out what was once feared in the same way as a traumatic neurotic dreams of his trauma, or as a child experiences pleasurably in play what he is afraid of in reality. (54)

Many such counter-phobic individuals may in fact achieve a measure of success in warding off their anxiety if they meet certain conditions, says Fenichel, and it is here that the ritualistic pattern of Joseph Smith, Jr.'s seductions must be examined most closely. The first such precondition is the transformation of passivity into activity or, in a sense, "identification with the aggressor." The counter-phobic person must actively seek out the situation repeatedly. The second is some form of protective or permissive promise from or to a trusted person, granted in either

---

[2] It is worth recalling the comment of Anna Freud in Chapter 3 that "[p]ain augmented by anxiety . . .[,] even if slight in itself, represents a major event in the child's life and is remembered a long time afterward, the memory being frequently accompanied by phobic defenses against its possible return" (53).

direction. The third precondition, if the early event was sadistic and/or sexual in nature, is that the promised protection is couched in terms that ensure that there will be none of the feared violence when the thing is confronted. And the fourth precondition is that the quest for the original feared situation must be carried out in order to become convinced that there really was no form of punishment in the situation after all. To live that experience and *not* to be punished is the goal of the counter-phobic attitude.

With this construction in mind, it would be useful to ask why there may have been for Joseph Smith, Jr. an apparent dissociated link between his childhood operations and his behavior toward women, his doctrine of plural marriage, and the entire ritualistic pattern of his sexual activity. It has been a major thesis of this book that Joseph's childhood trauma was for him a symbolic dismemberment trauma with powerful lasting effects on his personality and behavior. The counter-phobic construction seems to link the trauma to his sexual behavior.

Joseph shared his age-appropriate oedipal fantasy with virtually all other young boys. He did *not* share with other boys the gradual successful resolution of this critical dilemma, for his trauma instead appeared to dramatize to him the worst possible outcome in a graphic and indescribably painful morality play in his own bedroom. Joseph's dissociated "lesson" from this punishment, in simplest form, seems to have been that erotic fantasies may be met by severe punishment. As Shengold notes, "If the abused child's experiences are primarily those stemming from aggressive attacks . . . there is almost always a defensive sexualization of those experiences" (55). Eroticism would become for Joseph a "password" to dissociated fear of violence.

Joseph would attempt to conquer the fearsome eroticism directly by facing it down and confronting it again and again, each time gaining some measure of comforting reassurance that it really would not always result in that painful punishment. Even so, the fear would never go away—the childhood event with its triple repetition seems to have been too horrible for that. And, therefore, neither would the anxiety.

And then the worst really did happen. In the middle of a seem-

ingly gratifying series of erotic encounters, each presumably providing partial reassurance that there was no reason ever to have
feared any painful punishment (but never quite good enough to
have abolished that fear), the mob entered Joseph's Ohio bedroom after midnight to take their vengeance for those encounters. He reexperienced the pain, the hostile gang of "about a
dozen" men, the violent struggle, and the reappearance of the
surgeon's scalpel poised to rob him of the focus of his greatest
pleasure—all of which struck at the very core of the reigning fantasy of his earlier assault. "In the midst of the 'triumph' which the
counter-phobic individual can enjoy . . ." warns Fenichel, "un-
pleasure may break out if something occurs which seems to confirm the old anxiety" (56). If there had ever been a small chance
that Joseph's repetitive sexual conquests could have abolished
that old unmastered fear, that chance almost certainly ended on
a cold March night in Ohio in 1832. His counter-phobic behavior
would become a consuming fixture of his life.

Turning to Fenichel's four necessary preconditions for a useful counter-phobic attitude, it is reasonable to examine if and how
each was specifically elaborated by Joseph Smith, Jr. The first, the
frequent and active seeking out of the feared situation, is self-
evident. That erotic activity with women opened Joseph's "dissociated memory file" is revealed by the recurring dream of the
angel apparition with his drawn sword and the threat to the potency of Joseph's "Priesthood" unless he continued to take more
and more women at an ever-increasing rate. Joseph's passive fear
of eroticism had evidently been converted into an active and repetitive search for this very goal. The powerful counter-phobia
had seemed to overrule all of those futile rational brakes applied
to his behavior by the norms and taboos of societal custom, by the
wrenching suffering of his jealous wife, and by the clear and present danger to his own life and that of thousands of his loyal followers against ever more militant enemies. Like a cocaine addict,
Joseph Smith, Jr. seemed to have become a slave to his counter-
phobia.

Fenichel's second condition, the necessity for some grant of
"magical protection," is what sets Joseph Smith, Jr. off from lesser
religious figures. It shows, equally as well as does *The Book of*

Mormon, his remarkable creativity. The counter-phobic individual must secure from an outsider some "protective or permissive promise, actual or magical, before engaging in an activity which would otherwise be feared" (57). Or, alternatively, the counter-phobic person could demonstrate that he himself is protecting or pardoning another person. Out of this latter expression apparently grew Joseph's elaborate superstructure of men progressing to godlike status through their expanding personal kingdoms made up of families with offspring "as numberless as the stars in the sky"—all the result of numberless erotic experiences with numerous women (so numerous, in fact, that the act might one day be no longer fearful). And all of this occurring without the fear and guilt of rivalry for those affections—the final fulfillment of the oedipal wish.

But most important, the sexuality was *primary*; the eschatology flowed out of it merely as a by-product. Each woman would be granted the awesome protection of eternal glory in Joseph's grand scheme, ordered by a recurring dream of an angel whom he dared not disobey. No woman, even if already married, should suffer guilt or remorse in this grand design, for she would continue to perform her earthly duties to her husband even as she enjoyed preludes to that which was to be hers forever. She would one day enjoy with the prophet "Celestial Glory," the most exalted condition of the eternal afterlife, in return for so small an exchange as her consent in the periodic sharing with him of a small fearsome act. "God almighty bless you. . . .," Joseph assured young Lucy Walker. "It shall be that joy and peace that you never knew" (58). "Whatever God requires is right, no matter what it is . . .," he wrote to Nancy Rigdon, "right, because God gave and sanctioned by special revelation" (59). Joseph granted to each woman the very protection of God himself, as he "extended his arm" of permission on earth.

A special dividend of the protective and pardoning precondition of Joseph's counter-phobia was realized when he began to share the blessing of Jacob with the fraternity of his priesthood. He could then vicariously experience triumphs over his fear through identification with other men by "pardoning" their extramarital adventures, thus reassuring himself in the process. Their own delight in the practice seemed to make him buoyant. Indeed, after explaining the principle of "celestial marriage" to his twelve apostles for the first time, Joseph "reportedly clapped his hands and danced like a small child" (60). Elder William Clayton, Joseph's confidential clerk for the final portion of his life, swore in 1874 of his own recollections:

> After the revelation on celestial marriage was written Joseph continued his instructions, privately, on the doctrine, to my-self and others, and during the last year of his life we were scarcely ever together, alone, but he was talking on the sub-ject, and explaining that doctrine and principles connected with it. He appeared to enjoy great liberty and freedom in his teachings, and also to find great relief in having a few to whom he could unbosom his feelings on that great and glo-rious subject. (61)

This kind of compulsive unburdening by Joseph seems indicative of the magnitude of the driving force behind his dissociated con-flict. Indeed, with such focus on this idée fixe in his final years, one even wonders that there was time for thought of religion.

Aside from the single episode with Bennett over Nancy Rig-don's affections, there is in the available record a surprising pau-city of rivalry between Joseph and his priesthood over such matters. That Joseph made clear to his colleagues his own posi-tion in this hierarchy of husbands is nevertheless demonstrated unequivocally in the sworn statement of 18-year-old Martha Brotherton, a buxom English girl who was detained one after-noon by Brigham Young in the locked second-floor room above Joseph Smith's store in Nauvoo. After requesting her secrecy and trying to solicit the personal feelings of the young woman toward himself and inviting her to consider taking him as a husband, Young instructed her that

> Brother Joseph has a revelation from God that it is lawful for a man to have two wives; . . . and if you will accept of me I will take you straight to the celestial kingdom; and if you will have me in this world, I will have you in that which is to come, and brother Joseph will marry us here today, and you

can go home this evening and your parents will not know anything about it. (62)

When the shocked Martha did not agree to this plan, the President of the Council of Twelve Apostles locked her in the room. Her affidavit continues:

> He was absent about ten minutes and then returned with Joseph. "Well, Martha," said Joseph, "it is lawful and right before God—I know it is. Look here, sister, don't you believe in me?" I did not answer. "Well, Martha," said Joseph, "just go ahead and do as Brigham wants you to—he is the best man in the world except me." "Oh!" said Brigham, "then you are as good." "Yes," said Joseph. ". . . and if you will accept of Brigham, you will be blessed—God shall bless you, and my blessing shall rest upon you, and if he don't do his duty to you, come to me and I will make him—and if you do not like it in a month or two, come to me and I will make you free again; and if he turns you off I will take you on." (63)

This exchange conveys better than any narrative description the nature of the tolerance, the gratification, and the empathy of Joseph Smith, Jr. for his comrades' sexual triumphs, gained through his own permissive generosity. Such lack of all apparent jealousy (except for the figurative elbow-in-the-ribs to Brigham Young in the dialogue over their respective sexual prowess) supports the existence of the counter-phobic attitude in Joseph's behavior.

The third precondition cited by Fenichel for the success of counter-phobic behavior, that the promised protection be couched in terms that ensure the absolute impossibility of violence, was also fulfilled in Joseph's seduction rituals. Since Joseph correctly perceived that the real threat of a repetition of his childhood "punishment" existed only through the unauthorized disclosure of his sexual liaisons, every proposition was invariably accompanied by strict admonitions not to tell of the conversation. Assurances were demanded in each such encounter, often with the most pointed threats against the woman's reputation should she make any disclosure. Such pledges are described over and over in existing affidavits and statements about Joseph's advances toward women. The necessary granting of this assurance of confidentiality was, in turn, the protective or permissive promise given by the woman to Joseph, by which the counter-phobia was allowed to function. In May of 1842, Joseph addressed an overflowing assembly of the Nauvoo Female Relief Society with his wife in attendance:

> Put a double watch over the tongue . . . [You] should chasten and reprove and keep it all in silence, not even mention them again. . . . One request to the Prest. [Emma Smith] and society, that you search yourselves—the tongue is an unruly member—hold your tongues about things of no moment. A little tale will set the world on fire . . . lest in exposing these heinous sins, we draw the indignation of a gentile world upon us (and to their imagination justly, too). It is necessary to hold an influence in the world and thus spare ourselves an extermination. (64)

Thus arose the vast and complicitous web of deception within the Mormon community—the social extension of a very private problem of its inwardly frightened prophet. Following the damning disclosures of the expelled John Bennett in area newspapers around Nauvoo, for instance, Joseph persuaded thirteen leading elders to swear affidavits to the effect that Bennett's claims of an order of spiritual wifery were fabrications. A second similar statement that "John C. Bennett's 'secret-wife system' is a disclosure of his own make" (65) was signed by nineteen prominent Mormon women, including Emma Smith, Sarah Cleveland (a plural wife of Joseph), Eliza Snow (another plural wife), and others who were not at all ignorant of the true state of affairs. Newel Whitney signed the first affidavit, and his wife, Elizabeth, signed the second, although both had stood witness to their 17-year-old daughter Sarah Anne's marriage to Joseph less than three months before.

The pattern of vigorous sworn denial of polygamous practices, once initiated by Joseph in forceful terms, could not be abrogated, for those tiny few who ventured to speak traitorously to the contrary were subjected to such ostracism in the beleaguered community that the social consequences for them were crippling or worse. Joseph denied his unusual sexual behavior from the very beginning until that very denial would provoke his death. He had no choice. As his counter-phobia tyrannized his behavior, the dissociated corner of his mind knew of the unspeakable consequences that would ensue without the permissive protection of nondisclosure by all whom he had brought into that structure.

But the most telling part of the web of deception was that which Joseph himself exercised in violation of the inviolable rule that he himself had defined. The prophet had always maintained that, by definition, plural marriage could not be adulterous because one of the preconditions for its practice was that "the first wife shall put the hand of the wife-to-be into the husband's hand" (66). This principle was fundamental in his instructions to his twelve apostles and to the others whom he solemnly tutored in the blessing of Jacob. Prior to entering the Everlasting Covenant, each man must somehow convince his own wife of her duty to accept the new partner as Sarah had accepted Hagar. But despite many formal celestial marriages of his own, Joseph would demur to his troubled confidants' questions about Emma. "I've not yet received the feeling to tell her," he told Apostle Willard Richards on the day he married the wife of David Sessions. "I can't. . . . But when the time comes the Lord will tell me to go to her" (67). "Should I tell Emma now?" he mused later to Richards. "Something says wait" (68). The beautiful structure of the Everlasting Covenant, with gods and celestial kingdoms, had an elaborate superstructure fabricated through the dissociation arising from his trauma. The covenant had to be spelled out to justify his behavior, especially to others. His own conduct, however, permitted its own arbitrary exception.

Joseph's pattern of deception over his sexuality seems a prototype for such patterns in other important areas of his life, such as his money-digging activities, his acquisition and translation of *The Book of Mormon* plates, the arrangement of witnesses for the plates, and some economic and banking practices not described in this book. In each case there was an underlying conflict that drove his behavior in compulsive and repetitive ways in a futile attempt to resolve that conflict. When that behavior conflicted with the rules of the real world in some incompatible fashion, Joseph would be forced to choose between them. It was characteristic of Joseph Smith, Jr. that he would tenaciously stick to his nonrational justifications, often reacting with hostility to those who defended the world of the rational and legal. That he usually held the loyalty of family, friends, and followers in the face-offs was testimony to his genius, charisma, creativity, and charm. Joseph was very trusting of his own feelings and inner drives—so much so that he would follow them even when they conflicted with such traditional societal rules as honesty and compassion. He believed in the preeminent reality of that which he felt within, and he would be guided by these perceptions to the end.

The final condition for the success of a counter-phobia, the quest to demonstrate that there never really was any reason to have feared punishment for the thing in the first place, was manifested by Joseph in his collection of "trophies" at ever-greater frequency. The first group of plural wives is perhaps the most significant from the standpoint of understanding the origin of Joseph's counter-phobia, since it is the least encumbered by secondary circumstances. As nearly all of the women of this group were already married, Joseph's overt behavior closely parallels the oedipal triangularity of his childhood fantasy. Each of these women would be "rescued" from her rivalrous husband. For the same reason, the more prominent or more powerful-appearing to Joseph was the husband, the greater would be the wife as a trophy and the greater the reassurance against the feared consequences. This may help to explain why one of very earliest plural wives was the remarried widow of the famous anti-Masonic martyr William Morgan, who earlier had played such a powerful role in the fabric of *The Book of Mormon*.

It also helps to explain why Joseph had audaciously sought consent from most, if not all, of his twelve apostles for his own spiritual wifedom with each of their respective spouses (69, 70). In each apostle's awkward efforts to explain to his own wife the need for compliance, each had borne his own particular burden, but none was as eventful as that of John Taylor, whose wife, Leonora, lost part of her little finger in a pan-throwing rage when advised of her new spiritual duty. Whether by design or by second thought, Joseph rescinded this blanket request after submissive assent was granted in each case, announcing instead that the request was merely a test of faith for the Twelve. But he had at least experienced the triumphant benefit of the *fantasy* of having possessed the wife of each lieutenant and the sense of conquest in each submission. There seems no reasonable alternative explanation, other than the counter-phobic one, for making such a foolishly dangerous request of his most trusted associates.

Of course, as has been seen, Joseph's pattern of seducing predominantly married women broke of perceived necessity after Bennett's excommunication and deteriorated into a compulsive spiral of easier conquests of younger women. Presumably his increasingly dizzying rate of trophy-taking in the final year of his life compensated for the fact that he no longer experienced the danger of rivalry quite so keenly.

The end would come for Joseph when one of the most loyal of his apostles, William Law, finally went public with the entire polygamy story in the first and only edition of Law's fledgling newspaper *The Nauvoo Expositor*. The widespread disclosure of the prophet's sexual behavior to his own shocked followers and to the growing anti-Mormon community, voiced by such a trusted lieutenant, was so frightening to Joseph that his boldness outstripped any capacity of his ample legal apparatus to protect him. A blanket disclosure had been his worst fear all along. The mainmast of his counter-phobia had snapped, and his worst nightmare must surely follow. Bereft of rational control, in a fit of rage, he ordered the destruction of Law's press and the scattering of the type in the street.

Governor Ford of Illinois could neither stomach this attack on the First Amendment nor stem the public outrage on all sides. Joseph was arrested along with his brother Hyrum and incarcerated on the second floor of the jail at Carthage, more than 20 miles away. The brothers watched as their options for a favorable outcome rapidly vanished, one by one. The night before the mob came, Joseph had a nightmare that he related to a visitor the next morning. In it, the prophet was back on his Ohio farm viewing a scene of weeds and decay. He entered the weather-beaten barn, which he "found without floor or doors." Suddenly, a group of men burst into the barn, and their leader accused him of trespassing, "stating it was none of mine, and that I must give up all hope of ever possessing it." During the leader's tirade, Joseph first defended his claim to the property, but when the malevolent leader threatened him, Joseph relinquished his claim. But the leader would not be pacified, threatening Joseph "with the destruction of my body." Then "a rabble rushed in and nearly filled the barn, drew out their knives . . .," following which Joseph struggled out of the barn "about up to my ankles in mud," again bound by his legs (71).

His last dream would seem like so many before it in recalling the familiar imagery of the most dreadful event of his short life. The accusation of "trespassing" by a hostile male, the entry into the room of a large group of threatening men with knives, and the restraint of his legs seem self-explanatory. With the themes of sexual guilt and punishment pervading his real-life situation, it is hardly surprising that this dream should recur at the moment of impending final assault. Recurring dreams do indeed have antecedents in prior terrifying events of the real world.

When the vanguard of the drunken mob forced the cell door open the next afternoon, Joseph emptied his revolver into their midst. With his brother Hyrum mortally wounded on the floor beside him, Joseph turned to the window to see a hundred fixed bayonets brandished below in a final scene of his familiar nightmare. His hands were on the sill when two bullets penetrated his back. Freezing for a second he made the Masonic signal of distress, having embraced that movement in the final years of his life. He pleaded the accompanying Masonic appeal of extreme danger, "Is there no help for the widow's son?" and pitched slowly forward to the ground below. (One wonders if it was mere coincidence that this final Masonic utterance called forth that very triangle of fantasy around which so many of his life's conflicts had centered.)

There are several descriptions of what happened next. Joseph was indeed shot in the back four more times as he lay face down on the Illinois soil. One stylized story, probably apocryphal, describes a barefooted roustabout triumphantly lifting the lifeless prophet's head by the hair and raising his long knife to decapitate him. At that moment the orange sun reportedly streamed through a break in the storm clouds, terrorizing and paralyzing the assailant. The knife fell to the ground and the mob fled in panic, leaving Joseph's bullet-riddled body in a single piece. Although this final act of symbolic dismemberment would be unsuccessful—and probably never occurred at all—it mirrors the manner in which Joseph Smith, Jr. tragically viewed his own existence so much of the time, living under the unshakeable inner threat of the surgeon's imminent return and of dismemberment by the sword.

Notes

1. *Doctrine and Covenants*, Section 17, v. 1. Salt Lake City, Deseret News Company, 1880, p. 111.
2. Smith LM: *Biographical Sketches of Joseph Smith the Prophet and His Progenitors for Many Generations*. Liverpool, S. W. Richards, 1853 [reprinted New York, Arno Press, 1969], pp. 85–86.
3. Jessee DC: "Joseph Knight's Recollection of Early Mormon History." *Brigham Young University Studies* 17:29–39, 1976; see p. 31.
4. Cowdery O: Letters to W. W. Phelps (1835). Cited in Quinn M: *Early Mormonism and the Magic World View*. Salt Lake City, Signature Books, 1987, p. 124.
5. "Brother Winchester" letter, November 19, 1838. Quoted in Brodie F: *No Man Knows My History: The Life of Joseph Smith, the Mormon Prophet*, 2nd Edition. New York, Alfred A. Knopf, 1989, p. 237.
6. *Doctrine and Covenants*, Section 21, v. 1, p. 130.
7. Johnson L: "History of Luke Johnson (by himself)." *Millennial Star* xxvi, 1865, pp. 834–836.
8. Smith J: *History of the Church of Jesus Christ of Latter-day Saints*, Vol. I. Annotated by Roberts BH. Salt Lake City, Deseret Book Company, 1927, pp. 263.
9. Johnson L: "History of Luke Johnson (by himself)," pp. 834–836.

10. Young B: *Journal of Discourses,* Vol. 11. Liverpool, Albert Carrington and others, 1864, p. 5.

11. Johnson L: "History of Luke Johnson (by himself)," p. 835.

12. Ibid., pp. 834–836.

13. Smith J: *History of the Church of Jesus Christ of Latter-day Saints,* Vol. I, pp. 261–265.

14. Young B: *Journal of Discourses,* Vol. 11, 1864, p. 5.

15. Quoted in Kennedy IA: *Recollections of the Pioneers of Lee County, Dixon, Illinois, 1893,* p. 98. See also Newell LK, Avery VT: *Mormon Enigma: Emma Hale Smith.* Garden City, NY, Doubleday & Co., 1984, p. 43.

16. Terr L: *Unchained Memories: True Stories of Traumatic Memories, Lost and Found.* New York, Basic Books, 1994, pp. 77–78.

17. Terr L: *Too Scared to Cry: Psychic Trauma in Childhood.* New York, Harper & Row, 1990, p. 299.

18. Quoted in Howe ED: *Mormonism Unvailed.* Painesville, OH, 1834, pp. 261, 259.

19. Kelly EL, Braden C: *Public Discussion of the Issues Between the Reorganized Church of Jesus Christ of Latter-day Saints and The Church of Christ (Disciples), Held in Kirtland, Ohio,* . . . St. Louis, Christian Publishing Co., 1884, p. 202.

20. Lewis L: "Affidavit," in Howe ED: *Mormonism Unvailed,* p. 268. See also Newell LK, Avery VT: *Mormon Enigma,* p. 64.

21. Smith J: "Joseph Smith to Oliver Cowdery." *Latter Day Saints' Messenger and Advocate,* December 1834, p. 40. See also Vogel D (ed): *Early Mormon Documents,* Vol. 1. Salt Lake City, Signature Books, 1996, p. 42.

22. Cowdery O: Letter to Warren A. Cowdery, January 21, 1938. Huntington Library, San Marino, CA. See also Brodie F: *No Man Knows My History,* 2nd Edition, p. 436.

23. C. G. Webb [Joseph Smith's grammar teacher in Kirtland], quoted in Wyl W: *Mormon Portraits, Joseph Smith the Prophet, His Family and His Friends.* Salt Lake City, Tribune Printing & Publishing Co., 1886, p. 57.

24. See Newell LK, Avery VT: *Mormon Enigma,* pp. 64–66, 140–143, 212.

25. See Wyl W: *Mormon Portraits, Joseph Smith the Prophet, His Family and His Friends,* p. 60. See also Shook CA: *The True Origin of Mormon Polygamy.* Cincinnati, Standard Publishing Co., 1914, p. 130.

26. Brodie F: *No Man Knows My History,* 2nd Edition, pp. 457–488.

27. See Tanner J, Tanner S: *Joseph Smith and Polygamy: An Expose of Mormon Polygamy.* Salt Lake City, Modern Microfilm Co., 1966, pp. 41–47.

28. Quoted in Wyl W: *Mormon Portraits, Joseph Smith the Prophet, His Family and His Friends,* pp. 60–61. See also Shook CA: *The True Origin of Mormon Polygamy,* p. 130.

29. Quoted in Newell LK, Avery VT: *Mormon Enigma,* p. 65. See also Foster L: *Women, Family, and Utopia.* Syracuse, NY, Syracuse University Press, 1991, pp. 134–135.

30. Quoted in Foster L: *Women, Family, and Utopia,* pp. 134–135.

31. Pratt S: "Affidavit," May 21, 1886. Quoted in Shook CA: *The True Origin of Mormon Polygamy,* p. 132.

32. Littlefield LO: *Reminiscences of the Latter-day Saints.* Logan, UT, 1888. Quoted in Brodie F: *No Man Knows My History,* 2nd Edition, p. 478.

33. Church manuscripts, compiled by Herber AH. Photocopy, Reel E, 2:18. Brigham Young University. Quoted in Newell LK, Avery VT: *Mormon Enigma,* p. 125.

34. See Newell LK, Avery VT: *Mormon Enigma,* pp. 140–143.

35. Clayton W: "Affidavit," Salt Lake City, February 16, 1874. Cited in Shook CA: *The True Origin of Mormon Polygamy,* p. 84.

36. *Doctrine and Covenants,* Section 132, vv. 1, 4, 19–20, 30, 32, 34–35, 37–38, 41–42, 44, 48, 52, 54–55, 61–63, pp. 463–473.

37. Clayton W: "Affidavit," Salt Lake City, February 16, 1874. Cited in Brodie F: *No Man Knows My History,* 2nd Edition, p. 341.

38. *Salt Lake City Tribune,* 1886. Quoted in Newell LK, Avery VT: *Mormon Enigma,* p. 161.

39. See Newell LK, Avery VT: *Mormon Enigma,* p. 212.

40. *Saints' Herald* (Lamoni, IA) 26:289–290. Quoted in Newell LK, Avery VT: *Mormon Enigma,* p. 301.

41. Pratt S: "Affidavit," May 21, 1886. Quoted in Shook CA: *The True Origin of Mormon Polygamy*, p. 131.
42. Bennett JC: *The History of the Saints; or, an Expose of Joe Smith and Mormonism.* Boston, Leland & Whiting, 1842, pp. 243–244.
43. Jacob UH: *The Peace Maker.* Nauvoo, IL, 1842. Quoted in Tanner J, Tanner S: *Joseph Smith and Polygamy,* pp. 18–21.
44. *Times and Seasons* (Nauvoo, IL), December 1, 1842. Quoted in Shook CA: *The True Origin of Mormon Polygamy*, p. 80.
45. See Brodie F: *No Man Knows My History,* 2nd Edition, pp. 336–337.
46. Snow E: "Affidavit," August 28, 1869. Quoted in Shook CA: *The True Origin of Mormon Polygamy*, p. 133.
47. Snow ER: "Biography and Family Record of Lorenzo Snow." Salt Lake City, 1884, pp. 69–70. Quoted in Brodie F: *No Man Knows My History,* 2nd Edition, p. 303 (footnote).
48. Johnson BF: "Affidavit," March 4, 1870, Salt Lake City, in Jenson A: *Historical Record,* Vol. 6, Salt Lake City, May 1887. Quoted in Tanner J, Tanner S: *Joseph Smith and Polygamy,* pp. 221–222.
49. Johnson BF: Letter to Elder George S. Gibbs, October 1903, p. 14.
50. Lightner MER: "Affidavit," February 8, 1902. Quoted in Brodie F: *No Man Knows My History,* 2nd Edition, p. 444.
51. See Terr L: *Too Scared to Cry,* pp. 207–209.
52. Fenichel O: "The Counter-Phobic Attitude." *International Journal of Psycho-Analysis* 20:263–274, 1939.
53. Freud A: "The Role of Bodily Illness in the Mental Life of Children." *Psychoanalytic Study of the Child* 7:69–81, 1952.
54. Fenichel O: "The Counter-Phobic Attitude," p. 267.
55. Shengold L: *Soul Murder: The Effects of Childhood Abuse and Deprivation.* New Haven, CT, Yale University Press, 1989, p. 1.
56. Fenichel O: "The Counter-Phobic Attitude," p. 272.
57. Ibid., p. 269.
58. Quoted in Brodie F: *No Man Knows My History,* 2nd Edition, p. 478.
59. Quoted in Bennett JC: *The History of the Saints,* pp. 243–244.

60. Whitney HM: "Life Incidents." *Woman's Exponent* 22:39, 1882. Cited in Newell LK, Avery VT: *Mormon Enigma,* p. 98.

61. Clayton W: "Affidavit," February 16, 1874. Quoted in Shook CA: *The True Origin of Mormon Polygamy,* p. 85.

62. Brotherton M: "Affidavit," July 13, 1842. Quoted in Shook CA: *The True Origin of Mormon Polygamy,* p. 75.

63. Ibid., pp. 75–76.

64. Nauvoo Female Relief Society Minutes, 9th meeting, May 26, 1842. Quoted in Newell LK, Avery VT: *Mormon Enigma,* p. 115.

65. Smith E, et al.: Statement, October 21, 1842. Quoted in Shook CA: *The True Origin of Mormon Polygamy,* p. 62.

66. Noall CA: *Intimate Disciple.* Salt Lake City, University of Utah Press, 1957, p. 301.

67. Ibid., p. 317.

68. Ibid., p. 320.

69. Wyl W: *Mormon Portraits,* pp. 70–72.

70. Van Wagoner RS: *Mormon Polygamy: A History,* 2nd Edition. Salt Lake City, Signature Books, 1989, p. 41.

71. Smith J: *History of the Church of Jesus Christ of Latter-day Saints,* Vol. VI. Annotated by Roberts BH. Salt Lake City, Deseret Book Company, 1927, pp. 609–610.

Chapter Eight

Inalienable Rites

*B*aptism for the dead was one of many elaborate rituals established by Joseph Smith, Jr. for his church. There would be others, and some would be laden with imagery that is by now familiar. These metaphors would reappear in many disguises in the life of the prophet and his church. Among such examples are the temple rituals, many impassioned speeches, his ambiguous plans for his own succession, and lesser vignettes that punctuate the biographical record.

Ever since the days of the elaborate money-digging rites, the historical record demonstrates a veritable compulsion of Joseph to create repetitive ceremonies for occasions of mystery. As plans for his first temple were being fashioned in Kirtland, Ohio, Joseph searched the Scriptures to find inspiration for ceremonies appropriate to the grand edifice. As in several other religious sects of the frontier, he first settled on the New Testament practices of ritual anointing, bathing, and foot washing. Joseph wrote in his history:

On the 23rd of January [1833], we again assemled in conference; when, after much speaking, singing, praying, and
praising God, all in tongues, we proceeded to the washing of
feet (according to the practice recorded in the 13th chapter
of John's Gospel), as commanded of the Lord. Each Elder
washed his own feet first, after which I girded myself with
a towel and washed the feet of all of them, wiping them with
the towel with which I was girded.

But Joseph betrays a most revealing mixture of metaphors as
he continues:

I then said to the Elders, As I have done so do ye; wash ye,
therefore, one another's feet; and by the power of the Holy
Ghost I pronounced them all clean from the blood of this
generation; but if any of them should sin wilfully after they
were thus cleansed, and sealed up unto eternal life, they
should be given over unto the buffetings of Satan until the
day of redemption. (1)

The religious rite of foot washing has represented humility,
homage, purification, and service since its ancient origins in the
arid cultures of Asia and Africa (2). But Joseph's introduction of
a representation that the practice was somehow related to the removal of blood is indeed an innovation, especially as that blood is
in some way related to misconduct. Prior to Joseph's pronouncement, blood had never played any role in the rite in all of its long
multicultural history. His own modification of the metaphor is understandable, especially in its anatomic proximity to his own
wound. So is Joseph's relating the cleansing away of the blood to
a pledge not to engage in forbidden acts any more, under the
threat of the most terrible punishment at the hands of the evil father himself.

In addition to foot washing, Joseph added the familiar anointing with oil and finally the sacrament of "lustration" in which the
entire body was bathed. The historical record available to the public is murky concerning Joseph's earliest ceremonies of washing
or any of the transition stages into the elaborate ritual of the temple into which it would ultimately emerge. It is widely known,

however, that adaptations of the ceremonies of Masonry contributed substantially to the content and complexity of the rituals.

In contrast to his earlier incorporation of the prevailing anti-Masonic sentiment into *The Book of Mormon* in the late 1820s, Joseph had reversed course and heartily embraced this movement in the early 1840s. Although actually taking its origins from no earlier than the thirteenth century, Masonry was falsely rumored to have been in full flower since the days of Solomon. The link to this earlier temple-builder, whom Joseph perceived to be an adopted ancestor and a like spirit in sexual privilege, had been more than a little appealing to the prophet. Joseph established the Nauvoo Lodge on March 15, 1842, with John C. Bennett as secretary. After being installed as a first-degree Mason on the first night, Joseph rose immediately to the highest degree only 24 hours later. He persuaded many of his priesthood to follow suit, and the lodge grew to nearly 300 members in a short time (3).

By May of 1842 Joseph had achieved the full fusion of Masonic ceremony with the religious rites of his own temple. In truth, he had merely grafted Masonic ritual onto his own. He had justified his action by instructing that Masonry as then practiced was but a kind of incomplete bastardization of the Solomonic order. By linking his priesthood to the Masonic rites, he would be able to institute "the ancient order of things for the first time in these last days" (4) as the genuine Hebraic endowment. This was to have been made possible, according to Joseph's followers, because

> [t]he angel of the Lord brought to Mr[.] Joseph Smith the lost keywords of several degrees, which caused him, when he appeared among the brotherhood of Illinois, to "work right ahead" of the highest, and to show them their ignorance of the greatest truths and benefits of Masonry. (5)

Joseph began to imbue his church with the language and world view of the Masons. On May 1, 1842, he recorded the following:

> I preached in the grove, on the keys of the kingdom, charity, &c. The keys are certain signs and words by which false spirits and personages may be detected from true, which cannot

be revealed to the Elders till the Temple is completed. . . .
There are signs in heaven, earth and hell; the Elders must
know them all, to be endowed with power, to finish their
work and prevent imposition. The devil knows many signs,
but does not know the sign of the Son of Man, or Jesus. (6)

Joseph found Masonry to be a wonderful framework over
which to drape his ideas, his icons, and, indeed, those many smoldering issues that troubled his sleep. In ways that recall the early
incantations of his father into the necromantic arts, Joseph seems
to have become enchanted by the Masons' possession of certain
"keys" in the form of words and signs by which they could distin-
guish between true and false spirits. He thus encouraged members of his priesthood to become Masons in order that they could
know all the signs (7).

But merely becoming a Mason would be insufficient. Joseph
took those keys, signs, costumes, secret names, passwords, oaths,
and ceremonies and built his Nauvoo temple around them. The
fullness of these promised mysteries of the ritual, he proclaimed,
could not be fully conferred until the temple's completion. Second to baptism for the dead, these rituals became an additional
motivating force to encourage his followers to complete construction of the temple in Nauvoo. In truth, some Mormon temple rites were first performed in Nauvoo's Masonic Temple (8). In
addition, some of the characteristic symbols of Masonry soon became familiar icons of Mormon architecture and design, including the beehive, the All Seeing Eye, the clasped hands, the phrase
"Holiness to the Lord," the square and compass, and the juxtaposition of sun and moon and stars (9).

The temple rituals in their final form are the highest representation of Joseph's sublimations as a playwright. In them can be
seen many of his familiar dissociated images taking form in the
symbols and characters of these dramatizations. But these tab-
leaus are distinct only in their complexity from those he created
on midnight treasure-digs in the farms of upstate New York.
Watching them, participating in them, and directing them with
a certain intensity, Joseph repeatedly acted out his conflicts
through ritual in a driven effort to expunge his lingering pain.

The temple rite was actually a kind of morality and fertility pageant built out of some primitive themes. Originally restricted only to men at its founding in 1842, the ritual would be opened to women before Joseph's death two years later. The elaborate ceremony began with washings and the donning of special white clothing, progressed through some symbolic dramatizations in which those going through the ceremony participated, and concluded with "endowments."

The initial washings and anointings, apparently always performed with and by members of the same sex, were quite "raw," in the words of those who first disclosed the nature of the Nauvoo ceremonies. I. M. Van Dusen, a participant in the early ritual and author of the first public description of the events, detailed his observations of this stage of the ceremony:

> There is a variety of ceremony going on in this room, some of rather too delicate a nature to speak of, as this work is designed to be read by all classes of both sexes. I am, however, divested of the remainder of my clothing, which leaves me in a state of perfect nakedness, and placed in a horizontal position in a bath of water that has been prepared for that purpose, and am washed from head to foot. (10)

The entire body, including the genitalia, was vigorously scrubbed by an officiant. As Van Dusen described his washing:

> All this time I am rolled and tumbled about from one side of the bath to the other. Head a part of the time under the water, half strangled under a considerable excitement, not knowing what is coming next. (11)

The first words of the ceremony went to the heart of Joseph's early surgical trauma: "Brother, having authority, I wash you that you may be clean from the blood and sins of this generation" (12). That which followed accompanied the ritual washing, one body part at a time, and resembled to some degree a fertility rite:

> I wash your head that your brain may work clearly and be quick of discernment; your eyes that you may see clearly and

discern the things of God; your ears that they may hear the
word of the Lord; your mouth and lips that they speak no
guile; your arms that they may be *strong to wield the sword*
in defence of truth and virtue; your breast and vitals that
their functions may be strengthened; your loins and reins
that you may be fruitful in propagating of a goodly seed;
your legs and feet that you may run and not be weary, walk
and not faint. (13) (emphasis added)

Anointing with oil followed the washing and was accompanied by
a similar pronouncement.

Following the ritual cleansing, a white garment was applied.
Initially (at least according to John C. Bennett) the garment was
a sort of shirt that was worn only at the ceremony and was then to
be hidden away as a kind of talisman for protection against "Destroying Angels." Soon, however, the garment was altered into
a one-piece suit resembling long underwear, described by Joseph
as identical to that worn by Adam and Eve in the Garden. Joseph
directed the cutting of the original garments and insisted that they
be bound with "turkey red," but ordered the red binding to be removed after a time. Again, the function of the garment was protective, for it required wearing at all times to preserve the wearer
from danger.

The garment was ritually slashed in places by the officiant at
the ceremony. A pattern of the Masonic compass was initially slit
into the garment in the region of both knees, but the region was
later changed to the left breast. The slash across the knee was
originally so deep that it drew blood and healed with a noticeable
scar. However, objections from some of the women participants
brought this practice to an end. An additional slash across the ab-
dominal portion of the garment symbolized the disemboweling
that would accrue to anyone who might choose to reveal the secrets of the ritual.

The thematic material resembling Joseph's operations is
abundant in this initial purification rite. The fundamental metaphor is unmistakably that of washing away blood and putting on
white garments. One remembers his mother's description of the
terrible event:

> ... and oh, my God! what a spectacle for a mother's eye!
> The wound torn open, the blood still gushing from it, and
> the bed literally covered with blood. . . .
>   . . . but when the act was accomplished, Joseph put upon
> a clean bed, the room cleared of every appearance of blood,
> and the instruments which were used in the operation re-
> moved, I was permitted again to enter.[1] (14)

The washing of the genitalia by the officiant, ordinarily a societal taboo, is also understandable when one remembers the sexualized nature of Joseph's fantasies. And finally, the sword is
figuratively placed into the hand in a reenactment of the childhood trauma in the spoken charge to the participant.

The whiteness of the garment—its freedom from the frightening redness of the blood—is apparently the most important
feature of the apparel. The red color with which Joseph had the
original design trimmed seems proof positive of the significance of the metaphor. His decision much later to remove the
red binding (as in the viewing of clean bedclothes long ago) is
perhaps a recapitulation of a wish-fulfilling fantasy, as evi-
denced by the protective effect that is somehow bestowed by
the whiteness. The white garments of this temple ritual (like
the frequent similar metaphor in *The Book of Mormon, Doctrine and Covenants,* and Joseph's many speeches) thus seem
to have functioned as a kind of repetitive plea from within, be-
speaking an unresolved mortal fear that the pain might one day
return. And who would bring that pain? As John Bennett describes, it was the same one who inflicted it in the first place:
the Destroying Angel, undoubtedly the same apparition that
appeared to Joseph with the drawn sword to order him to institute plural marriage. Like Lady Macbeth's ritual, the lustrations
of the temple represent Joseph's futile, repetitive efforts to wash

---

[1] It is significant that Joseph would remove his own garment before starting
for Carthage, where he knew he would be killed. Although he gave the
reason at the time that "he did not want his garments to be exposed to the
sneers and jeers of his enemies" (15), it is perhaps just as likely that the
certain prospect of seeing his own blood on the white garments might
have been too painful a reminiscence.

free of blood the evil that had produced his unshakable guilt in the first place.

If there were any doubt about the specificity of this part of the temple ritual toward the childhood operation, it should be dispelled by the final act of violence: a slash across the knee so deep it drew blood and left a permanent scar. The convenient disguise of this act as a supposed symbol of the Masonic compass is an example of the way in which Joseph merely grafted Masonic symbols onto the ritualistic displays of his own inner conflicts. The deep slash inflicted on the participant by the officiating elder (Joseph) is but another example of "the need to take on the attributes of the tormentor and turn on other victims the abuse that was suffered" (16). Joseph would by this violent dramatization compel others to experience what he had suffered so long ago. It is worth noting that the choice of "knee" rather than "lower leg" for the slash is likely related to the fact that the type of osteomyelitis that young Joseph suffered typically attacks the very highest portion of the tibia just below the knee joint.

What is to be made of the reference to a slash across the garment covering the abdomen and the threat of disemboweling is not at all clear, but it is worth remembering that Joseph's mother's account of Alvin's death mentions an immediate autopsy and examination of his intestines. If this did indeed happen, it would certainly have been performed where the patient died—in this case at the Smith home—as was the custom of the day. This could not have been a pleasant memory for Joseph, especially in view of previous discussions of this matter.

The second part of the temple ritual was an allegorical drama in which Joseph reportedly played the role of God, and his brother Hyrum, that of Christ. Following an opening scene of the Creation, the participants proceeded into a tableau of the Garden of Eden. There they watched the entry of a priesthood actor playing Lucifer, who carried a cane, sometimes wore a long tail, and wore a sort of Masonic apron, sometimes decorated with crossed crow-quills, sometimes with a serpent, and sometimes with pillars surmounted by balls (17). As Lucifer tempted Eve and the familiar story unfolded, the dialogue proceeded in part as follows in at least one published version:

EVE: Who are you?

LUCIFER: Your brother.

EVE: You my brother, and come to tempt me to disobey Father!

LUCIFER: Oh, I said nothing about Father. Here, take some of this fruit: it will open your eyes.

EVE: But our Father said in the day we ate thereof we should surely die . . .

EVE (*to Adam after eating the fruit*): Adam, here is some of the fruit of that tree; it is pleasant to the taste and will make you wise.

ADAM: I shall not partake. Don't you know our Father commanded us not to touch the fruit of that tree?

EVE: Do you intend to obey all Father's commands?

ADAM: Yes, all of them.

As the familiar story reached its climax with the banishment from the Garden, the dialogue between the gods continued:

ELOHIM [*the supreme god*]: Let Adam be cast out of the garden and cherubim and a flaming sword be placed to guard the way of the tree of life. [*A sword is waved through the curtain.*]

[*Eve . . . looks up at the sword and crosses over to Adam and places herself on his left hand.*] (18)

The dramatic sequences of this ceremony are vintage Joseph Smith, Jr. Their principal motif is that of a young, innocent, honorable hero (Adam) who faces the dilemma of good-father versus evil-father through the *splitting* device discussed in conjunction with the story of Laban. The evil-father Lucifer carries a cane and wears a tail, both transparent symbols of the source of his power (along with other similar symbols of crow-quills, serpents, and pillars surmounted by balls on the apron). The paternal relationship with the good-father is openly spoken in the dialogue where the term "Father" is unmodified as a reference to God ("tempt me to disobey Father," "our Father commanded us," "obey all Father's commands"). The "flaming sword," with its connotation of the threat of searing pain, is given greater attention in the ceremony than in Genesis. In its position as guardian of the lost paradise, it is a familiar symbol. The sword forbids access to the most desired object of the young hero, as proscribed by "Father." In contrast, the final dramatic act fulfils a wish as Eve looks at the mighty paternal sword waving through the curtain and then *chooses* Adam, crossing the stage to forswear the triangular relationship in the young hero's favor. The eternal oedipal theme, subtle and mysterious in Genesis, is graphically, blatantly, and grimly expressed in Joseph's dramatization. Driven by the lingering conflict within, the sexual theme is again accompanied in ritual by the imminent threat of destruction and dismemberment.

After the initial dramatization, the participants in the temple ritual were robed and instructed with a secret name, grip, and sign regarding the Aaronic priesthood. Adam admonished them not to disclose any of the ceremony at the threat of throat-slashing. There followed a ceremony of satire about other faiths, during which an actor says of Lucifer, "Why, he said we should have no more Apostles and if any should come along professing to be such I was to ask them to cut off a leg or an arm and put it on again, just to show they had come with power" (19). Additional priesthood tokens were bestowed as the participants pledged not to disclose the secrets at the risk of having "our breasts cut open and our hearts and vitals torn from our bodies and given to the birds of the air and the beasts of the field" (20).

The remainder of the ceremony was a progression to glory. First was a pledge of sacrifice and recitation of the law of chastity, differing by a significant word or two between the sexes, pledging to "covenant and promise that you will not have sexual intercourse with any of the opposite sex except your lawful husband (wife or wives) given you by the holy priesthood" (21). There followed a prayer, a lecture about temple rites, and further ritual communications. A ritual facing position between the participant and the Lord was assumed as the Lord whispered, "Health to the navel, marrow in the bones, strength in the loins and sinews, and power in the priesthood be upon me and my posterity through all generation of time and throughout all eternity" (22). Triumphal entry into the Celestial Room followed.

In this final part of the pageant the dismemberment threat, first expressed in the Garden of Eden scene, is expressed in even more explicit language in the bestowing of the tokens of the priesthood. The admonition accompanying the first token of the Aaronic priesthood calls forth the image of the nearly decapitated ghost Joseph had described in an early version of the first visit to Hill Cumorah (see Chapter 4), for the temple participants are warned "that our throats be cut from ear to ear and our tongues torn out by the roots." The second token of the Aaronic priesthood is accompanied by a less disguised reference in the warning of the "vitals torn from our bodies." The clergyman in the play could have asked for any of a thousand miracles, but for some reason the specific request was that ". . . I was to ask them to cut off a leg or an arm and put it on again," a request through which Joseph's preoccupation with dismemberment is once more revealed. And the Lord's blessing of "marrow in the bones" is self-explanatory as a further reference to Joseph's tragic trauma.

"The close affinity of religious and phallic rites is a commonplace in social history," Brodie wrote in 1945, "and Mormon ritual doubtless had its roots in the same unconscious drives that led the prophet into polygamy" (23). Indeed, it did—with the same angel, the anxiety over the same fearsome sword, and the same dissociated memories of the dreadful event in his childhood. Some themes are indeed universal in the minds of men, but those themes may become terrible tyrants if horrifying childhood experiences scorch hotspots into the mind.

There is a particular issue that matters very much to today's followers of Joseph's religion: the issue of the prophet's succession. It matters because there are today two sizable organizations, each of which claims Joseph's collective mantle. The Church of Jesus Christ of Latter-day Saints, headquartered in Salt Lake City, claims that Brigham Young was given instructions by Joseph to succeed him as leader of the church should he as prophet die. The Reorganized Church of Jesus Christ of Latter Day Saints, headquartered in Independence, Missouri, claims the office was bestowed by the prophet upon Joseph Smith III, his oldest son. Much of the legitimacy of each organization presumably hangs in the balance on this question.

Many historical facts surrounding the divergence of opinion are not in dispute. There were several claims upon the prophet role in the chaos of Nauvoo after Joseph's death in 1844. Most of these aspirants alleged legitimacy for this position by their own demonstrations of the sorts of revelations and mystical visions Joseph had displayed. In contrast, Brigham Young, with unmatched political acumen, claimed his authority through his presidency of the Council of Twelve Apostles as appointed by the martyred prophet. One by one, Young's rivals and their bands of followers left Nauvoo or were driven out. Young ultimately held the fealty of the major body of Mormons and led them on their monumental trek to the West, where he would maintain that loyalty in the building of the remarkable kingdom in the isolation of the Great Basin.

Joseph's family, meanwhile, detested Young and claimed that the leadership should pass to Joseph Smith III, only twelve years old at the time of the prophet's death. William Smith, the prophet's youngest brother, claimed he should hold the title in escrow himself until his nephew came of age. Several years hence and with the full support of Emma, whose scorn for Young was boundless, Joseph III at the age of 27 would accept the invitation of a sizable group of members who had not left the Midwest and would found the Reorganized Church. This organization, buttressed by Emma's straight-faced insistence, claimed that Joseph Smith, Jr. had never sanctioned or participated in polygamy in any way and blamed the practice instead on John C. Bennett and Brigham Young. The group also eschewed baptism for the dead and the temple rituals. The leadership of the Reorganized Church passed thereafter in a kind of royal succession from father to son until very recently.

The fact is that Joseph had actually intended that his brother Hyrum should lead the church if he himself should die unexpectedly and had taken some concrete steps to pave the way for this. In 1841 the prophet had delivered a revelation with this thought in mind:

> And from this time forth I appoint unto [Hyrum] that he may be a prophet, and a seer, and a revelator unto my church, as well as my servant Joseph,
>
>   That he may act in concert also with my servant Joseph, and that he shall receive counsel from my servant Joseph, who shall show unto him the keys whereby he may ask and receive, and be crowned with the same blessing, and glory, and honor, and Priesthood, and gifts of the Priesthood, that once were put upon him that was my servant Oliver Cowdery.[2] (24)

In the increasingly threatening days of 1844, Joseph made some efforts to maneuver Hyrum into a protected situation in order that his brother could assume the church leadership in the event of his own death. The prophet first tried to persuade Hyrum to take shelter in Ohio but was not successful. Later, in the desperate moments when Joseph was trying to decide how to respond to Governor Ford's summons to jail in Carthage, Hyrum again would not leave his brother's side. It is certain in retrospect that Hyrum would have assumed the presidency of the church had he not ridden with Joseph to Carthage (26). But expediency was one thing to Joseph; a grand plan for succession was quite another.

    There is evidence that Joseph envisioned that his own oldest son, Joseph Smith III, would follow him as president of his church. He had said as much when he had laid his hands on the boy's head in a jail cell in Liberty, Missouri, in 1839 and shouted, "You are my successor when I depart" (27). The boy was in his seventh year at the time.[3] A similar pronouncement was made in an outdoor sermon in the winter of 1844. On that occasion he called young Joseph to stand beside him and proclaimed, "I have often been asked who would succeed me as the prophet to the church. My son Joseph will be your next prophet" (28). Others remember

---

[2] Before Hyrum, Joseph had successively designated Sidney Rigdon, David Whitmer, and Oliver Cowdery in 1834 to fulfill the role (25).

[3] Since it is well known that troubled memories of childhood may be rekindled when one's own child reaches the age of one's trauma, the timing of the prophet's impassioned statement is perhaps more than coincidental.

an impression through the oral tradition that the popular boy was widely regarded as the chosen and expected successor of his father (29). However, no will by the prophet or other authenticated written documentation of such intent has been found.

From a pragmatic standpoint, however, Joseph clearly placed the authority for the functioning of his church in the hands of his Council of Twelve Apostles and its president, Brigham Young. During his increasingly preoccupied days of 1844, while he was trying to persuade Hyrum to leave town, Joseph feverishly instructed his apostles. One of the group described their being

> in council with Brother Joseph almost every day for weeks, said Brother Joseph in one of those councils, there is something going to happen; I don't know what it is, but the Lord bids me to hasten and give you your endowment before the Temple is finished. He conducted us through every ordinance of the Holy Priesthood, and when he had gone through with all the ordinances he rejoiced much, and said, now if they kill me you have got all the keys, and all the ordinances and you can confer them upon others, and the hosts of Satan will not be able to tear down the Kingdom as fast as you will be able to build it up; and now, said he, on your shoulders will the responsibility of leading this people rest. (30)

Another member of the Council wrote later that Joseph exclaimed to the apostles, "Upon your shoulders the Kingdom rests, and you must round up your shoulders and bear it, for I have had to do it until now" (31). The wife of one of the apostles similarly recalled a prayer circle she had attended:

> On that occasion the Prophet arose and spoke at great length, and during his remarks I heard him say that he had conferred on the heads of the Twelve Apostles all the keys and powers pertaining to the Priesthood, and that upon the heads of the Twelve Apostles the burden of the Kingdom rested, and that they would have to carry it. (32)

Since it appears that both arguments have merit, the claim on behalf of Joseph Smith III will be examined first. It should hardly be surprising that the prophet would follow the law of the firstborn. The powerful identification toward his own father and the displacement of that identification toward his own son should have overridden any other claim on the succession. As has been noted, this was a primitive issue with Joseph, one that accounted for his naming his son after himself and, perforce, his father. It was seen in his *The Book of Mormon* allusion through Joseph of the Old Testament to the "prophecy" of his own coming ("And his name shall be called after me; and it shall be after the name of his father"). As is well established, one available ego defense for resolving lingering male oedipal dilemmas is through having a son of one's own. As such, Joseph III, the prophet's firstborn surviving son, was a singular affirmation of his own manhood and the focus of transferred identification from his own father.

Joseph's sense of the propriety of lineage is demonstrated frequently in his structuring of the church and its appendages. The office of Patriarch (evangelical minister), for example, was designated thus by revelation:

> It is the duty of the Twelve, in all large branches of the church, to ordain evangelical ministers, as they shall be designated unto them by revelation. The order of this Priesthood was confirmed to be handed down from father to son, and rightly belongs to the literal descendants of the chosen seed, to whom the promises were made. This order was instituted in the days of Adam, and came down by lineage . . . (33)

Similarly, bishops were designated for the same sort of direct lineage in Joseph's ecclesiastical hierarchy. An additional example is seen in Joseph's revelation in 1841 concerning the construction of a boarding house in Nauvoo:

> And now I say unto you as pertaining to my boarding house which I have commanded you to build for the boarding of strangers, let it be built unto my name, and let my name be named upon it, and let my servant Joseph, and his house have place therein, from generation to generation; for this anointing have I put upon his head, that his blessing shall also be put upon the head of his posterity after him, And as I said unto Abraham concerning the kindreds of the earth,

> even so I say unto my servant Joseph, in thee and in thy seed
> shall the kindred of the earth be blessed. (34)

Judging from what is presumed of Joseph's view of the order of
the father-son relationship, especially as it pertains to the firstborn, the claim of Joseph III seems formidable.

But Brigham Young's claim appears equally strong. Young's relationship with Joseph had dated from 1832, ironically only two
days after Joseph III was born. Both Joseph and Brigham were Ver-
monters by birth, Joseph being a bit younger and taller than his
more muscular comrade. Young had been attracted to Joseph's
movement by his admiration for *The Book of Mormon,* and the political dynamism he brought complemented Joseph's mystical
creativity in a way that was greater than the sum of its two parts.
"The Lion of the Lord" became Joseph's strongest ally and his
most effective lieutenant. He had been Joseph's principal de-
fender among his own doubting people when the prophet had
been imprisoned in Liberty, Missouri, and had led the banished
and dispirited Mormons out of Missouri into Illinois with remarkable organizational and inspirational skill during that dark time.
Young's financial and business acumen had been responsible for
the creation of a measure of solvency in the undercapitalized early
days of Nauvoo and for the efficient emigration of thousands of
British converts with their much-needed financial assets. Left with
the stark choice between this natural, proven leader and his pu-
bescent son to take the reins of the church amid the murderous
hostility roundabout and the near anarchy within, Joseph could
not have hesitated.

But there seems to have been another connection between
the two men that gives the president of the Twelve Apostles a yet
greater claim to the prophet's mantle. Brigham Young seemed to
carry a measure of sexual aggressiveness that rivaled Joseph's
own. One gains a sense from studying the historical record that
Joseph shared his unorthodox sexuality more easily with Young
than with any other man. "I myself sealed dozens of women to Joseph," Young confided in 1866 (35). The list included the poet
Eliza Snow and other socially prominent wives. Young was among
the earliest of Joseph's confidants introduced to the new celestial

order of wives and its strongest proponent for the remainder of his life. The three-way conversation with Martha Brotherton quoted in Chapter 7 reveals much of their spoken and unspoken mutuality in the sharing of confidences in each other's sexual liaisons.

Joseph and Brigham shared both a strong appetite and a penchant for secrecy over their many sexual relationships. The apostle took forty-one wives before leaving Nauvoo, far more, apparently, than anyone else except Joseph himself. Young took another dozen or so later in his life and sealed himself to an additional 150 or so women who had already died. Although one non-Mormon actress, Julia Dean, apparently scorned his affections during her lifetime, Young sealed himself to her after her death, perhaps indicating something of the scope of his own sexual fantasies (36). As he aged well beyond middle life, he would proclaim, "I could prove to this congregation that I am young; for I could find more girls who would choose me for a husband than can any of the young men" (37). But despite this boisterous pride in his prowess, Young kept more than half of his sexual affairs and sealings entirely confidential, the record not being corrected until more than a century had passed. Was it in fact true, as alleged by John C. Bennett in his 1842 exposé, that there was more than one "class" of plural wife in Nauvoo? Whether yea or nay, it is clear that both Joseph and Brigham formally sealed socially prominent women to themselves on the record; other women they apparently took with less formality and greater secrecy.

One strains to search modern history for a parallel to the intimacies shared by these two men, presiding in their own world and claiming nearly absolute power in the sexual arena. In this new social order, where so much more time was needed than was available for social custom to adjust, power flowed to those who took it, and Joseph evidently admired the aggressive and virile posture with which Brigham approached his task. "[J]ust go ahead and do as Brigham wants you to," Joseph had told Martha Brotherton, "he is the best man in the world except me." A bold comrade such as Young would have been a comfort to Joseph in the fearful ambivalence of his own sexuality. Perhaps Young represented to Joseph the virile ideal he had for himself—the no-

longer-afraid sexual icon he could never become because of the
lingering dissociation of his childhood trauma. Joseph, in stark
contrast to many of Young's modern-day followers, would have
appreciated the small aging slab of marble yet adorning a grassy
hillside in Whitingham, Vermont, bearing the inscription,
"Brigham Young, Born on this Spot, 1801, A Man of Much Courage and Superb Equipment."

It would seem that both Joseph Smith III and Brigham Young
possessed ample claim upon the prophet's mantle. Each personi-
fied a major issue in Joseph's life—one his powerful father-son
identification, and the other his driven sexuality. The fact that
both issues had common roots in an incident in the prophet's
childhood bedroom does not help to resolve the argument. But
the lingering institutional debate between Salt Lake City, Utah,
and Independence, Missouri, is somehow appropriately symbolic
of the magnitude of the conflict that Joseph had to endure within
his own mind because of that very incident.

Countless other vignettes in Joseph's biographical record be-
speak his continuing internal struggle with his childhood trauma.
Most are to be found in symbols and in the imagery of his
speeches and writings. It is worth noting a few of the most con-
spicuous examples before concluding.

One thinks of the "whistling-whittling boys," a group of teen-
agers who occasionally appeared, as if from nowhere, in Nauvoo
when strangers in town posed threats to Joseph Smith or other
leaders. Each boy carried a short stick in one hand and a long and
very sharp knife in the other. Whistling casually, the boys would
saunter in groups toward the strangers, slicing shavings from the
sticks with long knife strokes. Words were never spoken as the
young men converged with knives flashing ever closer to the in-
terlopers. Few strangers failed to receive a clear message on
which they promptly acted. It is not hard to imagine Joseph's role
in conceiving and implementing this threatening little pageant,
patterning it after that most terrifying image beyond his conscious
memory. (One even wonders if Nathan Smith whistled while he
worked.) The imagery embodied in the knife strokes across

stubby sticks held just below waist level is barely disguised.

One remembers the famous watercolor painting of the last public address of the uniformed Lieutenant General Joseph Smith before the Nauvoo Legion. His unsheathed sword is raised on high as he proclaims:

> We are American citizens. We live upon a soil for the liberties of which our fathers periled their lives and spilt their blood upon the battlefield . . .
>
> Will you all stand by me to the death, and sustain at the peril of your lives, the laws of our country, and the liberties and privileges which our fathers have transmitted unto us, sealed with their sacred blood? . . .
>
> Come, all ye lovers of liberty, break the oppressor's rod, loose the iron grasp of mobocracy, and bring to condign punishment all those who trample under foot the glorious Constitution and the people's rights. [Drawing his sword, and presenting it to heaven] I call God and angels to witness that I have unsheathed my sword with a firm and unalterable determination that this people shall have their legal rights, and be protected from mob violence, or my blood shall be spilt upon the ground like water, and my body consigned to the silent tomb. (38)

As the sword is unsheathed, the blood is spilled, and the oppressor's rod is broken, so the dissociated conflict is also assuaged, but only partially.

And finally, one recalls with interest the Sunday in May, 1843, when Joseph ascended the pulpit and delivered one of his most famous sermons using a metaphor of himself on which none could improve:

> I am like a huge, rough stone rolling down a high mountain; and the only polishing I get is when some corner gets rubbed off by coming in contact with something else, striking with accelerated force against religious bigotry, priest-craft, lawyer-craft, doctor-craft, lying editors, suborned judges and jurors, and the authority of perjured executives, backed by mobs, blasphemers, licentious and corrupt men and women—all hell knocking off a corner here and a cor-

ner there. Thus I will become a smooth and polished shaft in
the quiver of the Almighty, who will give me dominion over
all and every one of them, when their refuge of lies shall fail,
and their hiding place shall be destroyed. (39)

The metaphor is the most splendid he ever uttered. Borrowing from the forty-ninth chapter of Isaiah, Joseph describes the
image of a craggy boulder being violently fractured and scarred by
downwardly crashing encounters until it is molded into an exquisite object of divine majesty and omnipotence—"a smooth and
polished shaft in the quiver of the Almighty." I have become, declares Joseph, God's own sword of Laban!

And with what or whom were those encounters? Joseph provides a litany of all the evil-father representatives he has faced during his lifetime, for that is how all those adversaries seem to have
been perceived, doctors included. And the result? That his own
"sword" has at last exceeded that of the evil-father. It has become
divine—greater than which no other man's may become, and so
large it cannot be taken away—the ultimate wish of the oedipal
boy.

That great polished shaft was taken out of metaphor by Joseph's
own followers in 1905 on the centennial of his birth. On that occasion the world's largest polished shaft of granite, one foot in
height for each of the prophet's 38½ years of life, was quarried in
northern Vermont, transported by rail and a twenty-two–horse
wagon, and erected at Joseph's birthplace in Sharon, Vermont.
The old sign, erected in the 1940s ("Visit the Joseph Smith Monument, World's Largest Polished Shaft"), has long since disappeared, but the shrine remains.

In concluding her unparalleled biography of Joseph Smith,
Jr., Fawn Brodie remarks, "Joseph's true monument is not a granite shaft in Vermont but a great intermountain empire in the West"
(40). I disagree. The empire was Brigham Young's. Only he had
the political skill to forge such a prosperous independent kingdom. Joseph had tried three times and had been ignominiously
driven out, along with his followers, in each dismal failure—in
Ohio, in Missouri, and in Illinois. His gift instead was in ritual and
metaphor, ever reverberating out of the stormy corners of disso-

ciation in his mind. The polished shaft rising from a wooded Vermont hillside is indeed the true monument, Mrs. Brodie. And Joseph Smith, Jr. would have loved it.

Notes

1. Smith J: *History of the Church of Jesus Christ of Latter-Day Saints,* Vol. I. Annotated by Roberts BH. Salt Lake City, Deseret Book Company, 1927, pp. 323–324.
2. See Fleming WL: *The Religious and Hospitable Rite of Feet Washing.* Sewanee, TN, University Press at the University of the South, 1908.
3. Smith J: *History of the Church of Jesus Christ of Latter-Day Saints,* Vol. IV. Annotated by Roberts BH. Salt Lake City, Deseret Book Company, 1927, pp. 550–552. See also Brodie F: *No Man Knows My History: The Life of Joseph Smith, the Mormon Prophet,* 2nd Edition. New York, Alfred A. Knopf, 1989, p. 280.
4. Smith J: *History of the Church of Jesus Christ of Latter-Day Saints,* Vol. V. Annotated by Roberts BH. Salt Lake City, Deseret Book Company, 1927, p. 2.
5. Burton RF: *The City of the Saints.* London, Green, Longman, & Roberts, 1861, p. 350.
6. Smith J: *History of the Church of Jesus Christ of Latter-Day Saints,* Vol. IV, p. 608.
7. See Goodwin SH: *Additional Studies in Mormonism and Masonry.* Salt Lake City, Grand Lodge F. & A. M. of Utah, 1927, pp. 33–35.
8. Temple Lot Case, U.S. Circuit Court (8th Circuit), Lamoni, IA, 1893. Cited in Brodie F: *No Man Knows My History,* 2nd Edition, p. 282 (footnote).
9. See Goodwin SH: *Mormonism and Masonry: A Utah Point of View.* Salt Lake City, Grand Lodge F. & A. M. of Utah, 1938, pp. 43–45.
10. Van Dusen IM: *The Sublime and Ridiculous Blended; Called, The Endowment.* New York, 1848, p. 7.
11. Ibid., pp. 7–8.

12. Paden WM: *Temple Mormonism: Its Evolution, Ritual and Meaning.* New York, A. J. Montgomery, 1931, p. 14.

13. Ibid, pp. 14–15.

14. Smith LM: *Biographical Sketches of Joseph Smith the Prophet and His Progenitors for Many Generations.* Liverpool, S. W. Richards, 1853 [reprinted New York, Arno Press, 1969], p. 65.

15. Huntington OB: "History of the Life of Oliver B. Huntington." p. 406. LDS Church Archives. Cited in Newell LK, Avery VT: *Mormon Enigma: Emma Hale Smith.* Garden City, NY, Doubleday & Co., 1984, p. 189.

16. Shengold L: *Soul Murder: The Effects of Childhood Abuse and Deprivation.* New Haven, CT, Yale University Press, 1989, p. 7.

17. Paden WM: *Temple Mormonism,* p. 16.

18. Ibid., pp. 17–18.

19. Ibid., p. 19.

20. Ibid., p. 20.

21. Ibid., p. 21.

22. Ibid., p. 22.

23. Brodie F: *No Man Knows My History,* 2nd Edition, p. 279.

24. *Doctrine and Covenants,* Section 124, vv. 94–95. Salt Lake City, Deseret News Company, 1880, p. 241.

25. Quinn DM: "Joseph Smith III's Blessing and the Mormons of Utah." *John Whitmer Historical Association Journal* 1:12–29, 1981; see p. 13. See also Newell LK, Avery VT: *Mormon Enigma,* p. 170.

26. *Scrap Book of Mormon Literature,* Vol. II. Chicago, Ben E. Rich, 1913, p. 461.

27. Wight L: Letter to the *Northern Islander.* Reprinted in *Saints' Advocate,* Vol. VII, September 1884, p. 478. Quoted in Brodie F: *No Man Knows My History,* 2nd Edition, p. 381.

28. Joseph III Letterbook No. 4, RLDS Library–Archives, Independence, MO. Quoted in Newell LK, Avery VT: *Mormon Enigma,* p. 170.

29. Brown H: *History of Illinois, From Its First Discovery and Settlement to the Present Time.* New York, J. Winchester, 1844, p. 489. See also Lee JD: *Mormonism Unveiled.* Omaha, F. H. Rogers, 1891, p. 155.

30. Hyde O: *Times and Seasons,* Vol. V. Nauvoo, IL, p. 651. Quoted in *Scrap Book of Mormon Literature,* Vol. II. Chicago, Ben E. Rich Publisher, 1913, p. 86.

31. Hyde O: *Times and Seasons,* Vol. V, p. 698.

32. Smith BW: "Affidavit," November 19, 1903. See also *Scrap Book of Mormon Literature,* Vol. II, pp. 86–87.

33. *Doctrine and Covenants,* Section 107, vv. 39–41, pp. 387–388.

34. *Doctrine and Covenants,* Section 125, vv. 56–58, p. 436.

35. Quoted in Dixon WH: *New America.* London, Hurst & Blackett, 1867, p. 225. Cited in Brodie F: *No Man Knows My History,* 2nd Edition, p. 334.

36. See Tanner J, Tanner S: *Joseph Smith and Polygamy: An Exposé of Mormon Polygamy.* Salt Lake City, Modern Microfilm Co., 1966, p. 48.

37. Young B: *Journal of Discourses,* 5, p. 210. Quoted in Tanner J, Tanner S: *Joseph Smith and Polygamy,* p. 48.

38. Smith J: *History of the Church of Jesus Christ of Latter-Day Saints,* Vol. VI. Annotated by Roberts BH. Salt Lake City, Deseret Book Company, 1927, p. 499.

39. Ibid., p. 401.

40. Brodie F: *No Man Knows My History,* 2nd Edition, p. 404.

Epilogue

All of the elements of religion converged in the tragic life of Joseph Smith, Jr. He suffered pain and humiliation, shed blood, and faced torment but transcended his personal struggle in metaphor. He died for having lived that metaphor to its fullest. None of his companions—nor he himself—understood the compulsion behind his unswerving course. But they followed and believed as much as with any Moses.

Only recently has appreciation been gained for the controlling power of prior emotional trauma, especially that of childhood. Although much of Joseph Smith's complex life will never be understood, there can be no question that the two major traumas he experienced—his own operations and his brother's death/exhumation—played primary roles in making him different from you and me. A fusion of both traumas was necessary for what he became. In the process he helped others deal with their own life struggles as he draped white and spotless garments over his own.

His religion surely did not arise in the serenity of a grove. It sprang out of the agony of an assault—"how great you know not." But as suffering is the cradle of creativity, Joseph's succession of personal tragedies produced a litany of religious thought that has inspired and comforted millions.

Whether this book has exaggerated or understated the roles of Joseph's traumas in his tragic life is open to debate. But the fact that he found the means to confront the residua of these lingering troubles is the source of his greatness. His internal compass and his courage to follow it changed the world.

Index